TANTRIC SEX AND KAMASUTRA POSITIONS

HOW TO SPICE UP YOUR SEXUAL LIFE AND
INCREASE INTIMACY. THE BEST AND
COMPLETE GUIDE TO ENJOY NEW
TECHNIQUES AND SEX GAMES IN
YOUR SPICY MOMENTS

Victor E.Sellner

© Copyright 2021 - All rights reserved.

This Book Includes

Book 1: 8 (FIRST PAGE)

TANTRIC SEX POSITIONS

INCREASE INTIMACY

AND YOUR OVERALL SEXUAL LIFE

Book 2: 110 (FIRST PAGE)

KAMA SUTRA SEX POSITIONS GUIDE:

LEARN HOW TO SPICE UP YOUR COUPLE LIFE.

FROM INTIMACY TO TECHNIQUES AND

SEX GAMES, EVERYTHING YOU NEED TO ADD

INTEREST TO YOUR RELATIONSHIP.

TANTRIC SEX POSITIONS

INCREASE INTIMACY
AND YOUR OVERALL SEXUAL LIFE

Victor E.Sellner

Table Of Contents

INTRODUCTION

I n the Tantric tradition, specific physical positions, which enhance the mind-body connection and promote more profound states of consciousness, are employed for sexual intercourse. The parts are believed to influence the development and progress of diseases. Most of these Tantric sex positions are based on the Muladhara or Base Chakra, located at the lowest point in the spine, representing the ground of their being or the concrete base the couple has in the physical world.

Like the other Tantric positions, these positions are part of the Tantric tradition, which can be traced back to the Hindu traditions' kama sutra and the Taoist teachings of China that both seek to harness sexual energy attain a state of physical, mental, and spiritual well-being.

These positions are designed to create a meditative and spiritual experience by prolonging the sexual act and merging with the sexual energy– for both the man and the woman. Although it is not physically possible for the man to satisfactorily indulge in both of these Tantric sex positions whilst being penetrated, he can however perform the same motions in a similar way to the woman, which benefits him greatly.

Tantric sex for the Tantric Buddhists focuses their attention on the Muladhara or Base Chakra. Tantra (Sanskrit, meaning "loom") is the term used to describe a yoga method that originated in ancient India and focuses on using sexual energy or desire to attain liberation and achieve spiritual interconnectedness. The word "tantra" itself means "to expand, to weave, extend, and be ingenious, skillful." Tantric Buddhism was brought to Tibet by the great Indian sage Padmasambhava, also known as Guru Rinpoche, in the 8th century. It is considered the most advanced form of Buddhism and is regarded as the core of Vajrayana Buddhism. Tantric Buddhists focus on touching and being touched in areas such as the genitals, which allows for more profound levels of intimacy and spiritual connection. This sexual energy is then purified to the central channel through meditation, enabling a state of ecstatic unity with nature.

The Hindu yogis most likely brought the physical positions and meditation techniques. Some contemporary has found that these practices influenced the early religious movements in Tibet like the great Mahayana Buddhist teachers. They were responsible for the introduction of Chorten, or mountain temples. From the local Hindu yogis in Western India, adept at Tantric meditation and other techniques, they introduced these practices into Tibet and China, which then spread abroad from the Himalayan region.

The Tibetan monks are commonly celibate, but the Tibetan lamas, the highest religious authority, are not required to be so. But at the same time, they maintain a vow of chastity as a sign of their spiritual commitment to superior beings. Currently, there are over 100,000 Tibetan monks who have taken full ordination within the Buddhist religion.

Bringing this into contemporary times, the Chinese Taoist teachings, which are hundreds of years old, teach that the man and woman are uniting in lovemaking embrace Yin and Yang's exchange or male and female energies. The joining of these opposite energies serves several purposes. First of all, it helps achieve a healthy body if the points are balanced, and secondly, it supports the attainment of spiritual freedom or enlightenment by the intensification of awareness. The sexual energy is conducted through the meridians, which are channels in the body that join the organs and the body's surface. The point is made to travel through the body, which allows for deep relaxation of the physical, mental, emotional, and spiritual organs. Achieving this heightened sense of awareness is the goal of this growth process into becoming a powerful being who can achieve real spiritual connection and achieve enlightenment.

CHAPTER 1:

WHAT IS TANTRA?

Tantra is a part of tantric sex, but tantric sex comes from both tantra and neotantra. Tantra is something that's found in advanced Hindu teachings, along with Buddhist and other Asian teachings. Tantra is something that's been around for many years, and it's an ancient ritualistic practice that involves practitioners, and close direction of the person who is guiding them, called a guru. Not as many people practice this form for a good reason.

The typical tantric sex that we know about that doesn't require a guru and isn't as ritualistic is neotantra. This was recently imported to the western countries, and it's only partially taken from the religious roots, so it's not as religious in practice as typical tantra. It's often called modern tantra or called "California tantra," but this is a derogatory term. This is often viewed as sexual practices together as a whole, not just sexual intercourse. This is typically used for more intimacy, and to help provide an orgasm that's more delayed and or powerful not just for themselves but also their partner.

However, there is also tantric sex within Hinduism, and there are a few interesting aspects of it.

Buddhism and Tantric Sex
Tantric sex was used in Vajrayana Buddhism, and this one is a very advanced form of Buddhism, but it still has 10 million adherents to it, and two schools mostly focused on this. You can

find this in Mongolia, China, Nepal, Russia, India, Tibet, and Japan for the most part.

One of the main goals of Buddhism, however, is to overcome your desire. This was the idea that the best way to achieve this was to experience passion, and from there, try to train it so you can control this.

His idea was that the people who were on his pathway would do this to attain enlightenment. They might be restricted for a while and practice tantric sex to experience the culture, rather than mere pleasure.

It did adopt the Hindu idea that the energy centers within the body, which are the chakras that are there, could be activated and released. The goal is to get the chakra at the crown of the head, which is where spiritual evolution is, and from there, transform your consciousness, and ultimately reach for nirvana.

The Buddhist traditions might use sexual yoga to magnify and move the energy that's innate within them. This does have orgasms, of course, but it doesn't have just pleasure-seeking ideas behind this. Often, the sexual energy is then deflected to the mystical channel that focuses on enlightenment rather than mere pleasure.

Of course, this practice isn't without danger s. Sometimes, you might use these techniques to achieve orgasm, or by getting the methods and sharing them with people who shouldn't know, that could result in mental illness, or you may have rebirth cycles in hell due to this.

Again, this tantric practice is ritualistic in aspects of putting your life in order and putting you in synch with nature as well. The idea behind this is to ritualize yourself from the moment you get up, during the day, as you go to bed, and when you're sleeping until you wake up the next day. You don't even have to use sexual yoga to practice tantra, but instead, you try to practice restraint and understanding.

What about NeoTantra

Neotantra is that hybrid of both of these, where it combines a lot of the tantra styles of both.

It's imported for the most part, and it uses the traditional yoga positions, along with meditation and breath control. Still, it's taught outside of the Hindu religion and culture, and you don't have to be religious to do it.

Some people also incorporate massages into this, including tantric massages, bioenergetics, counseling, and sexual healing. You sometimes need to learn a course of study for a couple of these areas, but the average person can utilize tantric sex and benefit from it.

The goal that is sought by the person differs each time. Rather than just a state of tantric bliss like thin the other types of tantras, it pushes for more intimacy with one another, along with the delayed and amazingly intensified orgasm. The neotantra practice focuses much more on sex and having better orgasms, whereas the traditional tantra does not.

Tantra is excellent, but it's hard, and many times they focus much more on self-restraint. Neo-tantra is more about having fun, but they may not focus on the other tantric practices you might get from traditional tantra.

Neotantra has the connections to the new-age spiritual practices, but not always, but sometimes it does contain other forms of sacred sexuality too, and sometimes is used for advertising sexual education course s to others.

Some commercial sex workers will use this as a gimmick, too, to increases their sales. It does modify both the Hindu and the Buddhist tantra idea by getting rid of where the guru is involved and getting rid of the extensive and intensive meditation it otherwise calls for.

So why are people attracted to it? Well, I promise fulfillment and excitement while you stimulate your natural sexual impulses, along with the neurotic needs that you have emotionally, with a hint of spirituality. The cool thing about modern tantra is that you can learn all about all of the different ceremonies and philosophies, and they can be used to promote the tantra mentality.

The Kamasutra and the Anga Ranga are also a part of this in a sense, since it applies to these sutras, or positions, to accommodate for love along with sex that doesn't happen in traditional tantras.

The traditional tantra is excellent to understand and has some sexual elements at the core, but you need to realize that it's more than just that. It's just replicating the feelings of sex, love, and wellness in both a physical and spiritual form, bringing about a better understanding of the other person.

These different types of tantras are entirely valid, and neotantra is a good practice, but you should learn the difference between all of these. The tantra roots are ancient, and this older form is still handy. It's just adopted a modern concept for you to use.

CHAPTER 2:

HISTORY AND ORIGIN OF TANTRA

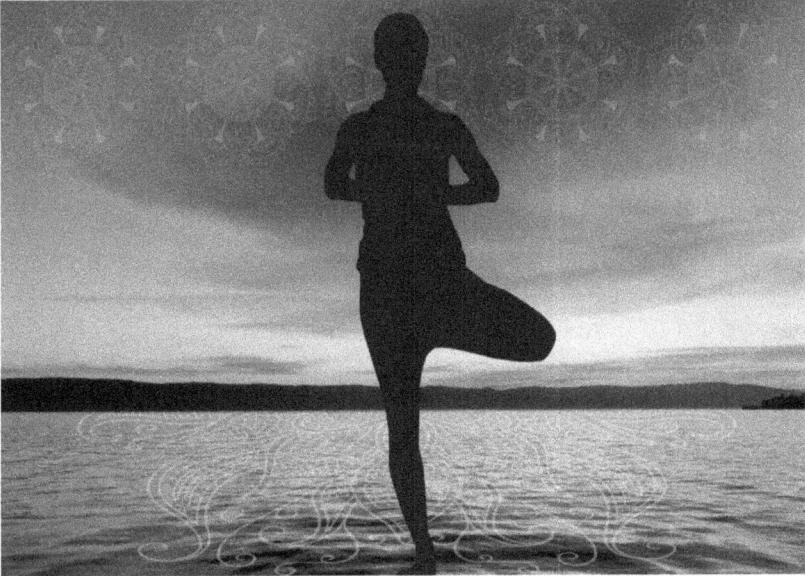

The original tantra, also called "red" or "left hand," is linked to ancient matriarchal societies and has female energy as its center. While the Tantra called "White" or "right-handed," created later due to Muslim infiltrations, derives from Indian patriarchal societies.

The difference between Red Tantra and White Tantra is radical. The second, White Tantra, is based on static and solitary meditations, while Red Tantra is a practice in which meditation is not just immobility and seriousness. In Red Tantra, meditation and sacredness are experienced in every moment of existence, through deep listening and attention to what is happening in us and outside of us. Reflection occurs while dancing, working, embracing, eating, drinking, playing, and talking. There is a lot of confusion about what Tantra is and, above all, a lot of targeted misinformation due to the persecutions to which the Original Tantra was subjected. Tantra carries the burden of false commonplaces, such as that of free sex. Unlike other disciplines that have been less polluted, Tantra is for many a kind of Yoga practice; for others, an orgiastic approach and for still others a religion.

The Origin of Tantra

According to the almost unanimous opinion of scholars, the archaic nature of Red Tantra dates back to pre-Vedic cultures, to the very beginnings of Indian history, identifiable with the Harappei, Sindhu, and other Dravidian populations which developed their civilization in the Indus valley. According to some, in the third millennium BC, these populations were widespread in a vast territory from Spain to the Ganges valley. Their precursors had settled in the Indus valley in Mehrgar, starting from 7000 BC, and their traces can be found up to 5500 BC.

Dravidian populations, therefore, appeared there around 6000-5000 BC, had their apogee between 2300 and 1300 BC., and disappeared, rather quickly, in 100 years between 1900 and 1800 BC. The disappearance's reasons were attributed in the past to invasions of the Arii population from the north. Today there is a tendency to attribute it instead to a tectonic movement that caused the Aravali hills in northern Rajastan to rise, depriving the river that supported the Dravida civilization (the Ghaggar-Hakra) of most of its tributaries.

The Harappei population showed a significant interest in the arts and well-being. Theirs was a matriarchal society, the most critical central monument of their city. It was a large swimming pool; the water element was fundamental in their organization, and there has already been a bathroom in every home. The woman was at the center of culture, focused on the mother goddess. The female figure dominated the sanctuaries and, with open arms and legs, offered herself to adoration. The Harappei used to keep a large bed in the center of the essential room in the house and practiced Tantra. Their religion was closely connected with the body, well-being, and sexuality.

It can be said that Red Tantra is the expression of all those practices, which also include sexuality. Red Tantra contains methods carried out in groups, including contact and "vehiculation" through the senses.

In the centuries following the birth of Tantra, in India, due to the Islamic invasions, the original Red Tantra was officially suppressed and forced to transform itself into an occult school. Today we know it as Tantra Yoga, and it has completely lost its peculiarity of a concrete approach to sexuality, typical of the original Tantra.

In practice, the White Tantra is a Red Tantra but censored by all those practices that moralists could understand as unbecoming. Today the White Tantra, which is, therefore, a mystification of the original Tantra, is used in the West for commercial purposes. Almost all Tantra schools practice White Tantra and therefore do not teach Tantra.

Authentic Tantra is the way of reconnection with one's self. It is the way; that of discovering our genotypic sexual energies that are manifested through the knowledge and practice of the Original Tantra.

The Tantra Texts

The Tantras are a series of texts of Central Asian origin (India, Kashmir, Bengal, Orissa, Assam, Kerala, Indus Valley, etc.) like the collections of the Puranas or the Vedas, but which manifest themselves in the manner of esoteric texts divine revealed and are often written as if they were the gods Shiva and Shakty (and their emanations) in-person speaking and are part of the Hindu Texts Agama.

The origin of the Tantras is pre-Vedic, which is much older than the texts on which Hinduism and the Vedas are based, and originates from the ancient matriarchal peoples and, in general, all the collections of Hindu texts are deeply influenced by the Tantra. No Hindu and Brahmin ritual does not have its roots in Tantra.

The Tantras were transcribed long after their birth, as previously the tradition was handed down only orally from master to teacher, from teacher to teacher. In fact, in Tantra, unlike Hinduism, the teachers could be men or women. Starting from about the VI AD instead, the written transcriptions of many Tantras begin to appear.

Tantric texts have more than one reading and can be experienced at different levels of intuition. According to the Tantric tradition, a text can confuse or illuminate. Tantric texts often speak by aphorisms (sutra and karika) and often then generate immense commentaries that explain aphorisms that can sometimes be difficult to understand.

The term Tantra, linked to the ancient texts, was then translated also to indicate the Spiritual Experiential Way that follows these ancient teachings.

More than 500 existing Tantras are known which belong to different initiatory ways or lineages. Many of them have never even been translated from Sanskrit. Other tantric texts have been lost, and it is not known what they handed down. It is said that the books reached a considerable number of 14000 volumes. So, the panorama of tantric initiatory texts is very vast, and not all Tantras treat themes equally according to the lineage to which they belong. So, this also generates some confusion regarding the teachings. Some Tantric Texts can be of a few pages, others of thousands of pages. It should therefore be understood that different teachings are grouped under the word Tantra, although on many points, many Tantra essentially agrees. It cannot be said that the various tantric texts contradict each other, but that they simply give certain importance more to one aspect than to another. Some Tantras favor the transmission of the concept of presence, others of the concept of the body, others concerning sexuality. A generally shared aspect is the "freed in life," that is, the unnecessary need for countless reincarnations to dissolve Karma. In fact, in tantra, it is indicated that by following certain rituals or teachings, it is possible to dissolve the karmic knots quickly, soon arriving at a knowledge of oneself also through the experimentation of eros and sexuality in the encounter between Shiva and Shakti and in any case following a way away from the renunciation of the body. The revelations of the Tantras are considered superior to the Vedas because they are much more effective in the liberation of men and lead them faster to a higher stage and are more suitable for the current cosmic era, the Kaliyuga. Tantra considers the Vedic texts to be valid, but on a lower level as basic general rules, but which are then integrated by higher and esoteric specific tantric teachings. Tantric texts do not address the renunciation ascetic of the world, but on the contrary, they address those who live in the world, together with others, without going away or dedicating themselves to asceticism.

How did Tantra Arrive in the West

In conjunction with the sexual liberation of the 60s and 70s and the emancipation of women, some scholars and philosophers began to talk about Tantra and trying to make it a practicable approach even in the West, made the rituals more agile and less blocking in the calculation of breath and holding of positions. Currently, emancipation allows women to get closer to the sexual world, although, in western society, it is still believed that sex is more masculine than feminine, and cultural heritage does not allow women to focus on that.

In the West today, Tantra aims to draw two maps, one that indicates how to make the sexual experience spiritual and how to unite the earth with the sky, in a terrain where separation and judgment vanish. A world, the western one, where there are no schools and traditions, and everything is to be invented and experimented with. In the West, the sexual sphere has been a world crushed for two millennia by taboos and religions, which often finds its only expression in private clubs or porn sites.

Tantra and the Way of Liberation

With all its erotic experiences, Tantra is nothing more than a tool that opens up internal physical, emotional, and energetic spaces and opens up to awareness. Tantra is, therefore, only Red Tantra. It is the way of liberation that opens up to the true expression of oneself, and that allows one to exit, both in the imaginary and in the real, from the dimension of the matrix in which sexual energy is mechanically channeled for improper purposes.

Sex and sexual energy are very different things. The idea of sex is what in the imagination has settled during education, stories, and commercial pornography, a program, therefore, but so rooted that individuals believe that it is precisely that pre-programmed way that sexual energy must be expressed. A program that is then gradually enhanced with the repetitive experiences that add up as memories.

The vital energy or commonly known as sexual energy (Kundalini), is instead what is the essence of the man at its origin; it is what we carry in our genes, but which, due to the education received in the matrix, is then unnaturally expressed in the facts.

Over time, with the help of religious morality, the matrix selected a sexual modality aimed entirely at procreation, therefore mechanical and centered on penetration and orgasm intended as a goal to be achieved; as if all the wonder of the contact between the bodies should be enclosed in the act of a few minutes, between the two genital organs. Many people believe they are sexually free because they do a lot of that mechanical sex, while in reality, they are just more slaves; slaves to a trap where true sexual energy is humiliated and crushed.

CHAPTER 3:

BENEFITS OF TANTRIC SEX

Y ou have encountered several benefits of practicing tantric sex. Yet, you will notice a vast difference in these new ones despite their interconnection. Those are not the only benefits you gain as you try tantric sex. There are more in wait for you.

1. **Expansion of Love Possibility:** With tantric sex, you are sure to expand the possibility of gaining love or deepening the love you and your partner have. It also would increase the spiritual connections that would allow you to adore your partner and still find yourself worthy of love.

2. **Health Rejuvenation:** The psychological and physiological effect that comes with tantric sex is sure to keep you in good health. They not only maintain good health but also help you in regaining poor ones.

    Take the breathing techniques you will learn later as an example. It will help you improve the way you breathe, thus giving your body more room to take in more air. This process will nourish your body tissues and muscles. Research shows that when we relax, meditate, or go on spiritual exercise, we are sure to improve our emotional and physical health. Spiritual people are sure to have lower blood pressure and less likely to be anxious or depressed. Not only those, but they will also have stable hormone levels. Invariably, their immune system will function better.

3. **Youthfulness:** Tantra allows you to tap into the fountain of youth. Since your body will not age quickly due to having healthy blood pressure, you are assured of the different things at your disposal to ensure you are looking young.

4. **Women Empowerment:** You were not waiting for that. But women are sure to suffer low-esteem about their bodies. Sometimes, they are careful about saying their sexual need because of this low self-esteem. But when you try tantric sex with your partner, the esteems of both individuals are skyrocketed because the body is treated with respect and honor. They feel desired and deserving.

5. **Empowers Men:** The two major problems faced with sex are the penis length and their longevity in bed. This has always ruined the experience because they are always looking inward instead of their partners' needs. They are also poor at pleasing women in bed because they focus on staying long instead of enjoying sex. When they don't focus on the women, they tend to displease the women more. Tantric sex is opening both parties to great satisfaction; thus, giving the man high esteem for his body.

6. **Great Sexual Satisfaction:** No doubt, sex has always left several people feeling they are not done. They want more and were left hanging in the balance because their sex was more genital-centric. The sexual connection didn't touch the heart or the soul. Tantric sex will help you make the heart feel the love and make the body feel more nurtured because of the soul connection you feel with your partner. As soon as the heart is fed with substantial sexual, the body and mind would enjoy the meal.

7. **Anxieties and Depression Alleviation:** One thing is sure, tantric sex will help in alleviating your anxiety and depression level. From statistics, several millions of people are battling anxiety and depression, which indicate that they suffer from such things as fatigue, restlessness, and sleeping/eating disturbance. You are sure to enjoy enormous positive energy from tantric sex that will improve the peacefulness of your body.

8. **Elevates Sex:** When sex is upped to a state of sacredness, then you are sure to enjoy a more luxurious dimension to it. This elevation would make regular sex seems wrong.

9. **Prolong Pleasure:** Tantric sex is simply upgraded lovemaking, which means there would be an extreme level of afterglow. This glow is sure to be on the increase because of the ejaculatory control and the way you directed your sexual energy in the spiritual manifestations.

10. **Healing:** As shown before, there are several ways tantric sex can heal you. Tantric sex will leave you with the feeling of being honored and respected in sex and life.

11. **Deepen Your Connection to Others:** Your self-esteem has been improved that you have little to worry about as regards yourself.

    This will make you stop worrying about yourself and start actually caring for people. Your connection to them will genuinely deepen.

12. **Be Relevant to the World:** Since you are no longer buried in yourself, your eyes are opened to the mysteries in the earth.

Your energy will alter the energy of the planet in a positive way. People are now feeling positive and are also generating good feelings about themselves.

CHAPTER 4:

The Tantra of Love

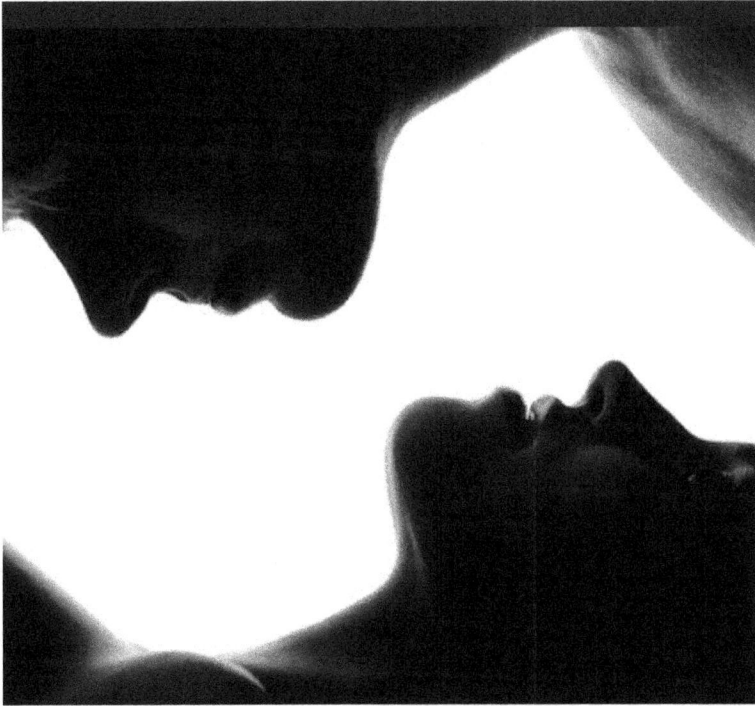

Tantra is the oldest sacred art of sexuality known to humanity and is still practiced to this day. However, the origin of the Tantra is not clear. There are different versions, including one that says Tantra is a disciplined Hindu system. Other historians say that Tantra comes from Buddhist monks. Still, others claim that Tantra was developed from rural communities in East India. There are other so-called experts who believe that yoga and tantra are one and the same. However, the key goal of yoga is to cultivate self-awareness and higher consciousness, while Tantra is about weaving and releasing the body. Considering the fact that most of the physically difficult positions of tantric sex are known from yoga positions, these experts have concluded that even if tantra is not yoga, it is modeled on yoga. The modern world knows about Tantra is that its most common form has retained some of the popular ancient writings, such as Kama Sutra (allegedly in Christ's day) and Anang Rank (a collection of erotic writings, first published in 1100 AD). A nobleman would be the author of the Kama Sutra. He saw life as involving dharma or a spiritual substance, artha or financial substance, and Kama, or sensual substance. The Kama is known as "enjoying the right objects by the five senses, aided by the mind and soul." Tantra may seem like the art of sexual pleasure, and Kama Sutra is a set of sexual positions. Kama's main goal is to cultivate love and develop worship and reverence for his partner's body. Looking at the tantric experience, it is easy to assume that you will have "great sex." However, if it is seen and experienced outside of the physical aspect (with clairvoyance), then it is, in fact, amazing dance and show of colors and energy, like the "epic experience of fireworks."

Opening of the Holy Chakra

To prepare for tantric sex, you must first learn to open the sacred chakra. To do this, follow the instructions below:

- Spend time near open waters and in the moonlight. It will help you feel and appreciate the healthy flow mechanisms in your own body.

- Try to surround yourself with beauty. For example, flowers, color, art, and music - or anything else that makes you happy and even more appreciative of your role in this world.

- Try using fragrances with sandalwood, musk, or ylang-ylang. They open the Holy Chakra more than any other perfume.

You can also repeat the following statements:

- I allow myself to enjoy my sexuality.

- I know that pleasure is an important and sacred part of my life.

- The opportunity to enjoy sex and sensuality brings me joy and nourishes my spirit.

- Let me fill my emotions well.

- My life is pleasant and graceful.

Tantric Sexual Experience is Divided into Three Stages
1. Physical

The main emphasis is on the physical pleasure that you feel at this particular time. Here are some of the ways that can help you experience physical tantric sex:

- **Stop Talking**

  Just get lost right now. Privacy is not just dirty conversations; Sometimes it's also about silence - how will you allow yourself to focus only on the moment and not think or talk about anything for a few minutes (preferably even longer).

- **Try to Slow Down**

  Undress. Focus on every part of the body, instead of being brutal right away. To enjoy the beauty of intimacy, you need to learn every part of your partner's body. You must appreciate the beauty of undressing and the joy of foreplay. Take your time - there's nothing wrong with that.

- ○ **Enjoy Sex without Orgasms**

  Sometimes you become intimate just because you can't wait for orgasm. Learn to enjoy foreplay and understand that even without orgasm, sex can be an incredibly beautiful experience for you and your partner.

- ○ **Give Him Life**

  This means that you also need to focus on breathing you and your partner. Hearing your partner's breathing sound can be sexy; you breathe the same air now and help you get lost right now.

  Improving this can make sex purely magical.

2. Emotional

Emotional tantric sex generally refers to a deep recall of love thoughts and the "worship" of another person's divinity.

This means that you need to create an emotional connection with the bed. Here's how you can work on it:

- ○ **Try to Say What You Want to Do**

  No, you don't have to do this when you are in bed and having sex, but you can talk about it during dinner and the like. Sometimes it's important to tell your partner what's going on - for example, the sexual fantasies you've always had - so that he/she can also think about how to implement them. Make sure it's a two-way street: learn how to give in to your partner's needs.

o   Recognize your emotional experiences with your partner.

Remember how you feel when you realize how much you love your partner. Try to delve into the deepest parts of the heart and find out what you really think about this person. Intimacy is not only about what you can physically share, but also how you know each other by heart.

o   Remember that none of you is perfect.

Sometimes you expect so much from your partner that you forget that he/she can fulfill your wishes only if you communicate properly. Make your expectations come true, and I don't want something you know you can't give. Always work to improve the communication skills and dynamics that both of you have.

o   Look into your eyes.

To be aware of a strong emotional connection, it is important to learn to look into each other's eyes during sexual intercourse. As you progress, you'll notice how different you feel about your partner compared to normal or normal sex.

- o Try to evaluate what you think about your partner in a sexual context.

  Are you delighted with the intimacy with your partner? What do you want to do with him and how do you think intimacy would improve your long-term relationship?

3. Spiritual

Spiritual tantric sex generally means feeling like one, associated with a "Supreme Being" or "God." And finally, you have a spiritual component that many people consider to be one of the most important parts of tantric sex. You can make it work like this:

- o Remember that sex is not just a relationship; it is a relationship between two people.

  In short, you both have to be involved in engaging in and achieving tantric sex. The powerful and ecstatic feelings that can be felt in the heart of a tantric sexual experience do not come from "forcing" an act or a deliberate attempt to manipulate another person. It must be possible to connect two people who trust each other and keep in touch (no wordplay is intended).

- o Go beyond self-absorption and narcissism.

  Always treat your partner honestly. Sexuality begins when you both reach maturity that is not based on narcissism or makes you feel less than you should. As a couple, you have a life together; it's important to recognize that this is the highest priority, even during sex.

o Get out of reality.

You don't need to think about all the problems you have in bed with your partner. Just think about the moment. Focus on leaving your problems outside your sexual experience. Basically, tantric sex can be a kind of meditation session if done correctly.

o Sex can be virtuous without prose.

Sex can be pure without one of you who could be a thriller. This happens when you both agree on what you want to do - and how you want it to happen.

o Tantric sex is also a form of prayer.

Why? Because it evokes the deepest parts of your soul and helps you keep in touch with another person. When you pray, it's not just about wishing what is good for you; he also cares about others and sex should be like that.

In addition to mystical and cosmic experiences, most tantric masters also seek deeper and more personal experiences with other people and the world in which they live. They believe that if there is a deep connection, then space previously seen between two people will be replaced by the light of the Supreme Being. They believe that this spiritual presence activates etheric energy between two people, "connecting them together" so that they can become one.

They believe that Tantra is actually a divine path that should be practiced with the greatest divinity and holiness. Tantra should be practiced as if one was engaged in a spiritual "ritual," and like most spiritual worship, it is inevitable to honor and recognize the Supreme Being. However, in this ideology, when you practice tantric sex, the deity is actually contained in your partner instead of a vague picture. Tantra is never an abstract form of sacred or sacred practice, but it is actually a practice in which experience with the Supreme Being is sent to the deepest areas of your senses. This does not mean, however, that you may not practice all other forms of worship or spirituality. The challenge of Tantra for all lovers is to feel, see, and hear the presence of the Supreme Being when they are united as one during tantric pranks.

Myths and the Truths about Tantric Sex and Tantra

Tantra is about celebrating sexuality and sensuality. It is a general misunderstanding that Tantra is based on sex. People, not fully aware of Tantra, know it from criticism.

Myth # 1: Tantric sex is about sex.

The truth: Tantric sex includes sex, but it's not just about genital contact. Tantric sex is about uniting souls, not just bodies. Genital contact or sex will only help increase the connection between souls. However, this is only possible if the couple feels at ease and are ready for this level of intimacy. Tantric sex includes various aspects that have absolutely nothing to do with sex.

Myth # 2: If you start practicing Tantra, you will simply give up pleasure.

The truth: This myth is loosely based on the previous myth. It's just a myth. Teaching Tantra does not include giving up sexual pleasure, as some yoga practices do. Tantra simply improves the level of pleasure. Tantric sex theory does not say that you must deny your desires. In fact, tantric sex encourages you to express your sexual desires freely. You don't have to imitate a yogi, sit cross-legged, or meditate for centuries to establish a connection with the Cosmos. Tantra realizes the importance of sex in the life of an individual and helps to use the undeveloped sexual energy present in the body to achieve happiness.

Myth # 3: Tantric sex increases sexual appetite and the need for pleasure that leads to business.

The truth: Tantric sex does not increase your sexual appetite and does not deceive you in the search for pleasure. Instead, it will help you control your desires and also help direct the sexual energy present in your body to a higher goal. Perhaps you were not even aware of your true potential. Tantric sex does not encourage having sex with multiple partners. This assumption has somehow reached many minds and is false.

Myth # 4: Turn you into a nymphomaniac.

The truth: Well, that's not true and it's pretty silly. Tantric sex helps to release all sexual energy present in the body, and also allows you to express yourself as easily as possible, but this does not mean that it will turn you into a nymphomaniac. However, the chances are that it will be misused. By exercising, you can control your desires and stop enjoying meaningless sex.

These common myths have spoiled the picture of tantric sex in the minds of the general public. This is not a taboo and should be practiced freely if you so choose.

CHAPTER 5:

Yantra

Yantra, in its literal translation from Sanskrit, means 'instrument' or a 'support.' In tantra practice, a Yantra is usually a geometrical design that is employed as a very effective tool to support the practitioner in meditative, contemplative, and concentration activities. Yantras represent the macrocosm in a microcosmic frame and acts as a gateway to and from the higher planes of consciousness. Yantras are all spiritually significant designs and every aspect has specific meanings pertaining to the higher planes of consciousness.

The Yantra in tantric practices behaves like a window to the universal divine being or the absolute one, as this power is many times referred to.

When you compel your mind to focus on a single design or object (the yantra in this case), the overwhelming mental chatter that clutters your mind is reduced. With practice, it is possible to eliminate mindless chatter in your mind completely. When the mind has achieved calmness and complete stillness, the yantra is dropped by the practitioners. A seasoned tantric practitioner only needs to visualize the yantra in his mind to reach a calm state of mind.

Yantras are usually designed symmetrically in such a way that the practitioner's eyes can be focused on the center. Yantras can be drawn on paper, on wood, on metal, or directly on the earth. They can also be three-dimensional objects. In India, the most famous one is the Sri Vidya yantra that represents the deity Tripura Sundari. This symbol is a microcosm of the entire universe and is used to remind the practitioners that there is no difference between the object and the subject.

Operation of Yantras

'Form energy' of 'shape energy' or the concept that every form or shape emits a particular energy pattern and frequency, is the basis of the operation of any yantra. Examples of such yantras that are seen even in Judaism and Christianity include the 5-pointed star or the Pentagon, the Star of David, the pyramids, the Cross, etc. These shapes are given different degrees of negative and positive power (or evil and good power). In Tantra practices, only those shapes that have positive attributes, and those with harmonious and beneficial energies are used.

When a practitioner focuses on the particular yantra, his or her mind automatically tunes in to the 'resonating' frequency or energy pattern of that yantra. Continued focus helps in maintaining and amplifying this resonating effect. It is important to remember that the energy itself as a result of the focusing exercise comes from the macrocosm and not from the yantra.

Therefore, yantras are instruments or tools that help us achieve resonance with a particular frequency from the macrocosm. The yantra facilitates the practitioner to 'tune in' to the desired frequency from the cosmos. It is possible to effectively use yantras to put the practitioner into elevated energy levels in the universe.

Types of Yantras Used in Tantric Practices

Unfortunately, the Western world is yet to understand the true meaning and the resonating power of a yantra. Many dubious tantric schools claim that they can draw Yantras by drawing on their imagination. This is not true. Every emotion has a specific yantra associated with it through the energy that its form and shape represent.

The traditional Yantras were not drawn from imagination but revealed through divine design and clairvoyance. Showing a new yantra to the world requires the limitless tantric powers of a true guru. Taking all and sundry 'designs' available on the internet as a yantra will only reduce the powerful influence of your tantric practice.

Yantras and mantras are connected because a particular yantra needs to be focused on by chanting a corresponding mantra. Here are a few yantras, along with a basic understanding of each of their resonance.

- The Dot or the Bindu – The Bindu represented focalized energy brought on by intense concentration. It can be seen as a deposit or reservoir of concentrated energy. In Tantric practice, the dot is considered to represent Siva Himself, the masculine source of all creation.

- The Triangle or the Trikona – This is a symbol of Shakti, the feminine source of all creation. A downward-pointing triangle represents the female sexual organ, the yoni, the Universe's supreme source. An upward-pointing triangle represents the supreme spiritual aspiration of being one with the absolute. Also, the downward triangle represents water which tends to flow down while the upward triangle represents fire which goes up always.

- The 6-Pointed Star of the Shatkona – Two triangles, one upward-facing, and the other downward-facing, superimposed over each other combine to form the shatkona, referred to as David's star in Judaism. This symbol represents the union of Siva and Shakti, without which there can be no creation.

- The Circle or the Chakra – Representing rotation, the circle is another commonly used symbol either by itself or as part of a more complex yantra in tantric practices. The process is also a very closely connected movement with spiraling movement, based on the evolution in the macrocosm. Moreover, the chakra or the circle is also a representation of the creative void and perfection. It symbolizes the wind element of nature.

- The Lotus Symbol – This is a symbol of variety (each petal is representing something different) and purity owing to the flower's ability to rise above a dirty pond to remain beautiful and pure.

- The Square or the Bhupura – Representing the element earth, the square symbol is usually the external contour of a yantra. Usually, a yantra uses the square as the contour and the dot as the center. This is the concept in tantra that the universe starts from the subtle (the dot – concentrated energy) and moves toward the gross (or the earth and life systems).

Many of the complex yantras also include other symbols such as arrows, swords, tridents, etc., representing the direction and purpose of the action of the form energy the yantra signifies.

How to Use Yantras in Tantric Practices

As already explained, resonance is the critical aspect of any yantra. The resonating effect of the yantra can be initiated and maintained by focusing on its image. The mind should be tuned to the resonating energy of the particular yantra for activation and sustenance of energy flow. Here are some instructions on the correct use of yantras:

- Hang the Yantra on any wall facing east or north ensuring the center of the image is in line with your eyes.

- When meditating, sit in a comfortable position that you are accustomed to.

- Inhale through the nose and exhale through your mouth in your natural breathing rhythm without trying to control your breath.

- Focus on the center of the yantra with as little blinking as possible. Keep the focus of your eyes on the center and watch the entire yantra as one.

- You can start with 5 minutes each day of this meditating exercise and then slowly increase the duration until you can do about half an hour a day.

- It is recommended that you aspire to achieve the levels of resonating energy that the yantra can deliver and your aspiration is bound to be fulfilled sooner than later.

- Seasoned tantric practitioners can reach such amazing depths in their focus that it is difficult for them to tell whether the yantra is within them or whether they are inside the yantra.

CHAPTER 6:

Mantra

With profound practices like yoga and contemplation winding up progressively prevalent, it appears as though everybody is discussing mantras. Be that as it may, what precisely is a mantra, and how are you expected to utilize it?

In our westernized, cutting edge otherworldly rehearses, "mantra" has progressed toward becoming as standard as "goal." But the two are entirely different. The word mantra can be stalled into two sections: "man," which means mind, and "tra," which means transport or vehicle. As such, a mantra is an instrument of the psyche — a ground-breaking sound or vibration that you can use to enter a secret government of reflection.

Like a seed planted with the goal of blooming into a beautiful lasting, a mantra can be thought of as a seed for invigorating an aim.

Yoga and Mantra
This mantra is utilized in quiet reiteration during development to help keep the mind centered. It has been said that in yoga, Asanas are stances of the body and mantras are stances of the brain. Mantras, when utilized in this design, are progressively similar to confirmations and help to keep you associated with a specific perspective.

Sanskrit and Mantra

Getting to the old foundation, all things considered, mantra, at its center, is the premise of every single religious custom, sacred texts, and petitions. At the point when deliberately picked and utilized quietly, mantras are said to be able to help adjust your intuitive driving forces, propensities, and burdens. Mantras, when spoken or recited, direct the mending intensity of Prana (life power vitality) and, in conventional Vedic practices, can be utilized to empower and get to otherworldly conditions of cognizance. As a profound practice, Mantra ought to be done all the time for a while for its ideal impacts to occur.

Toward the day's end, the mantra is intended to take you back to effortlessness. We live in such an unpredictable world that it is anything but difficult to lose all sense of direction in every one of the subtleties. Mantras can enable you to hover back to the oversimplified way to deal with life and spotlight those things that motivate you and satisfy you.

Reflection and Mantra

In this unique circumstance, mindfulness alludes to the capacity to focus on the decisions you make in your regular daily existence and perceive when something is not working so you can transform it. Numerous individuals face a great deal of pressure every day. Before the part of the bargain, prepared to crash. At that point, you rehash the cycle the following day.

Building up a day-by-day contemplation practice causes you to develop an increasingly present, quiet, and adjusted lifestyle, which swells out into each other part of your life. Mantras can help take you back to that current situation with the psyche.

You've most likely heard the word mantra previously. Be that as it may, what you can be sure of is this is an otherworldly practice, and it is as old as it is significant.

We will investigate what mantras are, the different ways they can be utilized, and best of all — how you can give them something to do in your very own life for mind-blowing mending, strengthening, and change.

All in all, what is a mantra? It is a word, sound, syllable, or expression that has an incredible vibration reverberation.

They are utilized in reflection, yoga, and in the otherworldly practices of Buddhism, Hinduism, and Jainism.

You can utilize a mantra to think about your vitality, open your chakras, and build up your mystic mindfulness. Otherworldly expressions, when opened, can raise your awareness. This training is so convincing and powerful. You have no clue where it could take you.

Personal mantra?

An individual mantra is an explanation that spurs and motivates you to be your best self.

With a personal mantra, you confirm how you need to carry on with your life. Also, it can help propel you to finish your objectives, both actually and expertly.

What Is Mantra Healing?

It has been demonstrated that reciting, music, and mantras strongly affect our cerebrum.

Mantras are fiery sound equations that moderate us down and permit us to see everything unmistakably. They give us a point of view.

Reciting quiets, the body and actuates various normal substantial capacities and procedures. It can likewise help in mending the psyche and body from addictions, such as smoking or liquor. Also, reciting can reinforce the resistant framework.

Reciting can lower pulse, lessen feelings of anxiety, increment hormone level execution, and abate nervousness and gloom.

Who might have imagined that this straightforward practice could have such control?

Yoga and Om Shanti

Om Shanti is maybe one of the most notable and open mantras utilized today. If you've at any point gone to a yoga class, odds are you've heard it.

All in all, what does Om Shanti mean? Indeed, there is a very immediate interpretation of Om Shanti. Om is not to such an extent as a word as it is a sound, an inclination, and a positive reverberation.

Om is said to be the sound of the universe. This single syllable incorporates the cycle of death and resurrection. Reciting the word Om carries you into an enthusiastic arrangement with the universe.

Anyway, shouldn't something be said about Shanti? Shanti is a Sanskrit word that signifies, "Harmony." Together, the Om Shanti importance is intended to pass on: Universal Peace.

It is regularly utilized as a welcome in yoga as a method for recognizing a kindred expert and wishing them harmony.

The absolute first mantras were utilized by Hindus in quite a while more than 3,000 years prior. A few hundred years after the fact, after Buddhism started to prosper, mantras began to be joined into their otherworldly practice as well.

Buddhist mantras depend on the heavenly lessons of the Buddha and the bodhisattvas. Here are three conventional Buddhist mantras you probably will not have known about previously:

- "Om Mani Padme Hum"

  This mantra is utilized in Tibetan Buddhism. That is to say, "I currently conjure the Universal sound, the gem, the objective of Enlightenment, love, and sympathy, Lotus shrewdness, and an unadulterated unified solidarity of insight with training."

  This is a routine with regards to empathy. It is utilized to look for and spread compassion for oneself as well as other people.

- "Om Muni Mahamuni Shakyamuniye Svaha"

  This signifies, "I summon the universal sound, Buddha-nature and the shrewd one, insightful one of the Shakyans, hail to thee!"

- "Om Vasudhare Svaha"

  Additionally, called the Buddhist cash mantra, it is utilized as a supplication to the bodhisattva of earth and wealth, Vasudhara. In Buddhism, Vasudhara is believed to exemplify the female soul and is the partner to the Hindu goddess, Lakshmi.

  Reflection mantras are a great method to build your care during contemplation. They serve as a point of convergence for your consideration, a similar way you may utilize a light, a photograph, or a statue.

There are many contemplation mantras you can access for nothing. The best part? They go about as a type of guided contemplation to enable you to remain grounded and present.

Here is a couple to kick you off:

- "Ham-Sah." Or, "I am that." This aide advises us that we are onlookers and separate from our human encounters and enduring.

- "Aham Prema." Or, "I am Divine Love."

- "Om Shanti, Shanti, Shanti." Or, "Genuine feelings of serenity, body, and discourse."

- "Om Tat Sat." Or, "All that is."

By what means can a mantra best be utilized?

Anyway, how would you utilize a reflection mantra? When you've chosen one, you'd like to attempt, locate a peaceful spot to start your contemplation practice.

When you are prepared, set the goal for your reflection. This is the place your chosen mantra will truly sparkle. Regardless of whether you'd like to ruminate for better wellbeing, more stillness, or only for a snapshot of harmony, set that aim before you start.

When you are prepared, start your mantra. You can say it so anyone can hear or in your mind.

Keep in mind; it is anything but a race. You can say it the same number or as multiple times as you'd like. Perhaps you have a specific number as a primary concern. Perhaps not. Essentially rehash your mantra gradually and with a goal.

Consider what your picked mantra implies. Harp on the individual words. Let the reverberation and vibration of every syllable ring.

This type of reflective practice is a ground-breaking one. Regardless of whether you've never attempted it, you will undoubtedly encounter transformative outcomes. Try it out.

Presently, in light of the fact that mantras are a 3,000 years-old profound practice doesn't mean they aren't similarly as viable today as they were in those days!

Mantras have changed throughout the years to oblige our cutting-edge frames of mind and recognitions.

A mantra shouldn't be articulated in Sanskrit to hold control. A mantra simply should be something that impacts you on a significant and individual level.

Mantras are frequently utilized in contemplation as an approach to remain engaged and focused. Be that as it may, you can utilize mantras from multiple points of view.

Print one out to set up on your divider. Record one on the network board at work. Slip a post-its mantra into your companion's handbag for an additional portion of motivation.

CHAPTER 7:

Yin & Yang

When you begin to follow the path of tantric sex, you begin to find a change in yourself. You find yourself changing how you view yourself and how you view the world. You find yourself looking at relationships that will last a lifetime. Through your journey, you will learn that every man and woman has a certain level of divinity in them. You will start to view sex as a sacred act instead of just a physical act. You will also learn to love deeper and find that you are soaring to different levels of bliss. You will only have a successful journey when you relieve yourself from any preconceived notions. You should not think of what you need to do and what your lover must do to please you.

You will learn the basic concepts of tantric sex and identify new exciting ways to live and love. The Yin and the Yang: Which is male and which is female?

You must be familiar with the stereotypes that men are from Mars, and women are from Venus. This implies that men are assertive and extremely powerful, while women are soft and fragile, who are only fit for nurturing. There are other stereotypes that men do not show any feelings whatsoever, while women have a plethora of emotion that is ready to unleash itself in a second. It has also been said that women do not take credit for the work that they do, since being outgoing is something only men are familiar with. Over the last few years, there has been a drastic change in the way men and women think. Tantric sex is a firm follower of the fact that men and women do have opposite characteristics. This is the elementary principle of the Tantra. The eastern theories claim that Yin represents feminism, while Yang represents masculinity. But there is no concrete proof that a woman cannot have Yang characteristics or that a man cannot have Yin characteristics. Rather than viewing men and woman as two entities, you should begin to focus on the energies. The Tantra believes in the amalgamation of these two energies.

Shiva and Shakti

The most common image of the Yin and the Yang is the Hindu divine couple Lord Shiva and Goddess Shakti. Lord Shiva represents the entire universe since he is considered the creator, and Goddess Shakti represents the root of all energy. The union of the two deities creates a longing in you and every other human being to be treated like a god or a goddess.

The male energy that is found in Lord Shiva represents ecstasy, while the energy in Goddess Shakti represents wisdom. This magical combination is what helps a person attain enlightenment. This perfect couple is always represented in numerous entwined positions – either dancing or embracing or standing together. There are other positions where Goddess Shakti is wrapped around Lord Shiva, with her legs propped around his hips. The dancing position by far is the most sacred since they can free their spirit, giving them a chance to attain enlightenment.

Understanding the Opposites

You may have made divisions amongst you and your partner. You first have to identify and understand these divisions to strike a balance between the opposite energies. There are quite a few stereotypical characteristics that you may relate to. You will have to identify those characteristics and make a note of them. You have to go from one extreme to the next. You should ask your partner to do this too. You will then have to see how you can embrace the extreme characteristics that you and your partner have. You have to identify how you can strike a balance between the polarities that exist between you and your partner. You will have to identify the Yin to your partner's Yang and vice versa.

You might now wonder if it is true that opposites attract. Sit back and think for yourself. You will be able to answer this question on your own. Try analyzing your past relationships. See how you and your partner were different from each other. Identify whether the differences were complemented by each other. This will help you analyze your future relationships as well.

My Partner is My Beloved

Tantra is not mad love but sacred love. You are honoring your partner and cherishing your partner while making love. You will shower unconditional love with your partner. When you are talking to your partner, use loving words like 'darling' or 'beloved'. You will find that those little words have aroused feelings of love within your partner. Call your partner with the aforementioned loving words when talking about him or her in public. You might find it strange to do so, but you will be sending out a message of love to the person you are speaking to.

The Desire Spectrum

You will find yourself with new views of desire. You may feel a desire every time you think of someone. You may comment on how you want a guy or how hot a girl is when you see them passing. You only feel these desires when you feel incomplete. Since you feel incomplete, you always want another person. You find yourself feeling needy and feeling wanted. But when you do get the person you want; you begin to want something more. You want someone prettier, more interesting, and sometimes someone richer. Through tantric sex, you will be able to detach yourself from superficial needs. This will help you create a healthier relationship with your partner.

You Feel Empowered to Say What You Want!

When you find yourself empowered, you can set boundaries both during sex and in life in general. You find yourself with a new level of self – esteem. In tantric sex, you own your body and your soul. When your partner wants you to enter you, he must ask for your permission. You should not be afraid and have to say yes or no as the situation demands. You have to stop and say that you do not want to be touched in a way that is not comfortable with it. You empower your partner when you speak the truth this way. You will be giving your partner the methods to use to please you. You have to be okay with how you are touched and how you feel.

CHAPTER 8:

Tantric Communication

D oes your associate virtually recognize how you want to be touched? How do you want to be loved? Imagine you may get precisely what you need in a mattress.

Before I knew approximately Tantra, I spent many a time mendacity with inside the fingers of my lover wishing he might do that or that. Thinking that if handiest he did this, then matters might be a lot higher for me. Conversely, I discovered myself questioning if he virtually favored what I gave to him if I turned into pleasurable his sexual and sensual goals. Obviously, the verbal exchange channels had been now no longer in particular open, subsequently we each wasted a whole lot of time questioning approximately the opposite's goals and wishes.

If we don't inform every different what we need and like, how are we able to in all likelihood anticipate our associate to satisfy our maximum mystery wishes intuitively?

Information Gathering in Tantra, one-of-a-kind strategies is used to open the verbal exchange channels and to create verbal intimacy in a context of considering. Being heard and listened to is as vital as sharing and telling our reality.

A Tantric verbal exchange starts off evolved with developing a sacred area. Sit down throughout from every different and proportion an include. Give every different compliment, bow right all the way down to your associate. With this exercise you're integrating a tantric mini-ritual into your lifestyles, making the verbal exchange exercise a unique occasion to be commemorated and cherished.

Now set parameters for the exercise. For instance, one character speaks, at the same time as the opposite listens for an agreed length of time, say ten mins. After the 10 mins, transfer roles.

The verbal exchange exercise usually revolves around a query. You could make up any query. For instance, "How do you want to be touched?" The speaker will reply to the query spontaneously. The listener will ask the query after which pay attention. If your associate runs out of answers, ask the identical query again. Note that this isn't a workout in communique approximately the subject, however, an excursion to benefit records approximately the opposite character and to exercise the artwork of listening.

The listener's function is to pay attention without a schedule and take with inside the records. By schedule, I suggest this – believe your lover tells you that she would love you to stroke her breasts in a total one-of-a-kind manner than you've got been doing when you consider that you acquire collectively. If you had a schedule at the same time as listening, you would possibly listen to yourself thinking, "How come she by no means instructed me this earlier than? Am I a total failure? Am I now no longer proper sufficient for her? Is she going to go away from me due to the fact I can't deliver her what she needs?"

If you had no schedule at the same time as listening, you'll take the records in and keep with the tantric exercise. And at the subsequent opportunity, you would possibly try and contact her breasts inside the manner she described. And you'll be pleasantly amazed at the aid of using her reaction!

At the quilt of the exercise, proportion an include and thank every different for generously imparting this treasured record.

In this Tantric verbal exchange, we discover ways to consider that the opposite character will deliver us what we really need due to the fact we created a secure and sacred area to invite for it

You might also additionally experience awkward answering an intimate query. Dare to speak! You are expressing yourself to your associate who desires to recognize all approximately you. Although awkwardness and shyness are a part of lifestyles, strive for something one-of-a-kind. For instance, you and your associate may describe how you want to be touched in very erotic terms. Or you may strive for the use of poetic language. This is one-of-a-kind out of your daily terminology. The humor and a laugh concerned creates a detail of lightheartedness that makes it clean to each specific goal and pays attention to them.

Loving feedback, another thing about Tantric verbal exchange, is the sensitive artwork of feedback. Imagine you're on a mattress together along with your lover and you're stroking his muscular shoulders. You suppose which you are doing a lovely activity and that he likes it very much. He lies there wishing you'll rub his shoulders harder. He receives bored stiff and all of a sudden informs you, "No, that's now no longer proper, rub my shoulders difficult as opposed to doing those feather-mild strokes." You at once flinch and don't need to head-on. You suppose you're now no longer proper sufficient that he doesn't like what you're doing.

Now believe this. He says delicately, "That felt very proper, my lovely beloved, however proper now I might pick a hint that may be a little bit firmer." You will experience mollified, preferred, and demonstrated for what you've got been doing, and can be handiest too glad to oblige and deliver him what he requests.

This is a great instance of tantric verbal exchange. Validate the one that you love earlier than you ask for something one-of-a-kind. Offer love and appreciation – she or he turned into doing his or her quality, after all – after which inform her or him what she or he should do to thrill you even greater.

Steve and I are surprised at what number of new matters we discover approximately every different in those verbal exchange rituals. We ought to have requested the identical query one hundred instances, and whenever the records we acquire from every different is one-of-a-kind and new. This is recuperation for each people and brings us nearer collectively.

Tantra is an effective transformational device this is a lot greater than intercourse!

There is a cultural craving for greater connection and intimacy in relationships. There is likewise a name for sacred and religious connections. People of all ages, genders, and sexual orientations are feeling the want for an area to connect to their frame, mind, and spirit in the community. Tantra gives methods to deepen your dating with yourself and others.

For people who are new to Tantra, it's far an exercise that mixes movement, breath, meditation, bodywork, and sound to help the powerful machine inside the frame, additionally called chakras, to open. This commencing lets in dormant power, additionally called kundalini, to transport up from the pelvis, alongside the spine. As this lifestyles-pressure power actions up the spine, it allows one to convert and heal. The recuperation includes loosening constrictions inside the frame that broadens for the duration of lifestyles. When the constrictions are loosened, one's real identity is revealed. Transformation takes vicinity, in addition to lifestyle shifts: sizeable bodily and emotional fitness improvements, new jobs, new or deeper partnerships, actions to one's dream location — those are simply a number of the results I actually have witnessed.

The goal of tantric practices is to increase one's frame and enjoy returned to the soul's authentic essence (called Purusha in Sanskrit): who you had been as a fetus, freed from strain or trauma, and who you're developing into as you end up unfastened. This is whilst we will come into our fullest potential, with acute attention and clean, loving reference to others.

On my very own Tantra path, and as a practitioner, I actually have held the area for lots to increase into their fullest selves. Over and over, I actually have visible that after chakras open, feelings stir. After all, they have become blocked or shriveled due to the fact one turned into now no longer covered or did now no longer experience secure being oneself. Contractions can end result now no longer handiest from a twist of fate or abuse, however additionally, from the consistent messages we acquire from society to be a person we're now no longer. Contractions inside the frame are an herbal reaction to shield your soul, which needs a lot to be unfastened to specific itself. However, the contractions have an effect on our cap potential to create and to permit pass of unsupportive habits, and additionally how we connect to others.

Inviting the chakra machine to open calls for braveness and readiness to take that leap, trusting that you may be supported and guarded as you heal and open to residing your real destiny.

Why are such a lot of humans turning to Tantra to clear up their dating challenges?

Tantra gives easy, beneficial verbal exchange strategies you could exercise and use at once for your everyday lives. Tantra can end up your new manner of relating — with a goal, care, and passion. We assist our college students to be sincere approximately what they revel in and what they don't in any given second.

Sexual abuse survivors and people with different sexual issues discover Tantra to be recuperation. We all want a discussion board to talk about sexual issues brazenly without shame and an area to research new methods of connecting in detail which are sacred, a laugh, and exciting.

Today, with the multiplied use of era for verbal exchange, each companion frequently retaining down complete-time jobs, and they want to coordinate parenting schedules, couples frequently glide apart. Tantra assists you in connecting, igniting a new passion, and considering why you got here collectively to proportion your lives.

Tantra-primarily based practices totally, just like the Divine Love Meditation below, assist domesticate intimacy with oneself and others.

Divine Love Meditation

Try working towards this meditation regularly, and word in case your verbal exchange transforms to a greater loving form — also, word how this fashion of verbal exchange impacts your relationships with others.

Tantra is ready to turn into embodied. Obviously, if you're analyzing this, you're embodied; you manifested in the world as a frame that homes your spirit. However, to be truly "embodied" to have intentional heightened attention to our very own presence. The frame is a doorway via which we will step into a fair extra experience of ourselves. By centering inside the frame, we open ourselves to what's past the frame, to a better vibration of our very own existence.

Some religious training takes an "out-of-frame" technique. Tantra rather invitations us to end up absolutely gift in the frame, to get entry to the deeper, non-bodily reality of who we're. It isn't approximately being greater bodily. It is ready centering ourselves with inside the remaining right here and now of our being.

How does this observe verbal exchange? Well, you recognize the expression "speak me heads?" It is used to explain TV pundits who're usually giving us their limitless opinions. In an experience, we're all "speak my heads." We speak from our heads. "I suppose, consequently I am," asserted Descartes returned with inside the sixteenth century. Identifying with our mind is certainly a not unusual place of self-referencing, of spotting who we're. Yet is it sufficient?

Thoughts are treasured and deliver a path to our lives. Emotions are an aggregate of our intellectual mind and the sensations or emotions we enjoy thru our frame. How mind experience in our bodies, what physical sensations we enjoy whilst we suppose or specific our very own or listen to any other's mind, and wherein we experience them, can deliver us effective clues to our internal reality. Thoughts and frame emotions feed on every different, impact every different. Thoughts generate emotions. Sensations that we enjoy with inside the frame cause mind.

CHAPTER 9:

Tantric Massage and Tantric Yoga

Massage is defined as a succession of strokes performed to promote muscular relaxation. However, tantric massage is more than that. The tantric touch stimulates, nurtures, and heals the body, the mind, the emotions, and the spirit. When done on its own, tantric massage can be an erotic experience. It can also turn into a therapeutic journey. When done before sex, tantric massage is a means of prolonging and building pleasure. When used as foreplay, the tantric touch relaxes your mind and your body so it becomes more receptive to your partner's gifts. It enables your sexual arousal to mount before it reaches its pinnacle. This way, your orgasms can become longer and more intense. Tantric sex is safe and healthy lovemaking. Some couples may feel pressured to engage in an intercourse in the early dating phase before they're emotionally attached or psychologically prepared. Using tantric massage as a pleasurable alternative for intercourse relieves them of this pressure. Tantric massage can be a fun and sexy way of getting to know each other deeper so that you'll have ample time to connect with each other emotionally. This way, once you finally decide to have sex, it becomes more meaningful and more satisfying.

Benefits of Tantric Massage
The busy and hectic life that we lead these days affects both men and women, and it causes several physicals, emotional, and even sexual disorders. Stress doesn't discriminate, and it

could trouble a person belonging to any age group, sex, or age. People need some relief if they want to enjoy their life to the fullest and they also have to replenish their strength to keep up with their hectic lifestyle. Massage can help in providing much-needed comfort and help you relax.

Among all the different types of massages that exist, tantric massage is gaining popularity. The main aim of a tantric massage is to provide you with a sensual experience that will also improve your health. Even though it is erotic, it helps the whole body to relax and has got several benefits.

o **Stress Buster**

Tantric massage can help you clear your mind, make your body feel light and help you relax. You can let go of all the tension and stress. Therefore, a session of tantric massage is recommended whenever you feel stressed. Stress is capable of making you feel miserable. If it isn't handled properly, it can cause several health problems as well.

o **Sex Education**

In many cultures around the world, sex education isn't adequate, and this leaves both genders unprepared for any sexual interaction or even sensuality. A tantric massage is the best way in which you can learn about your body. It provides you with a serial interaction that will help you to understand how your body works. It provides you with an insight into how your body works and the different parts that will make you feel other sensations. When you interact with your partner, it will be helpful to know what excites and pleases you both.

o **Premature Ejaculation**

Premature ejaculation usually tends to occur due to the pressure of performance. In most societies and cultures, men are considered to be the "doers," which puts an added pressure on them and causes them to ejaculate prematurely. Tantric massage helps in taking this pressure off them and lets them just enjoy the sexual act. When there isn't an expectation of them to perform well and without any specific goal in mind, men can perform well sexually. This will help in rectifying the problem of premature ejaculation. Tantric massage will help in teaching you to enjoy the moment, and during intercourse, it would also improve a man's ability to hold off his climax for a while longer. It is all about drawing out the pleasure to make the experience more intense.

o **Orgasm in Older Men**

As time passes by, and while the body starts aging, the body's hormone levels tend to decline and because of this older men feel little or even no sexual arousal, which means that they aren't capable of reaching an orgasm. Tantric massage can be beneficial for older men. This sensual massage helps in stimulating their senses and also helps in the production of the sex hormones and thereby helping them deal with problems like erectile dysfunction and the lack of achieving an orgasm.

o **Women and Sex**

In most cases, women don't enjoy intercourse. This could be caused due to various reasons ranging from their lover's inability to please them or even their lack of knowledge about their body. Women are sensual creatures, and it takes them a while longer to achieve an orgasm. Most might not even be aware of their bodies or what they like and dislike. Tantric massage will help them in understanding their bodies and their needs better. It will help them in deriving greater pleasure and even sensuality during any form of sexual activity.

Tantric massage helps in awakening your senses. It is sensual. We tend to perceive the world around us through our senses, and the awakening of the senses sharpens this perception of ours. Tantric massage is a therapeutic massage that has various health benefits. It can help relieve body pains and aches, stimulate your immune system, and increase your fertility. Many women can't orgasm, and tantric massage helps integrate your mind and body thereby facilitating their ability to reach an orgasm. Tantric massage tends to be empowering on various levels regardless of the characteristics of an individual. Tantric massage also provides the greatest form of relaxation and pleasure for your mind, body, and soul without having to reciprocate. Tantric massage involves the massaging of all the parts of the body. Having one's genitals massaged is quite a fulfilling experience. It also helps in creating a conscious connection between all the areas of a person's life. A massage without any expectations is quite a liberating experience. Tantric massage helps let go of the illusion of separation that exists and remedies this divide in every individual's life. It can also pave the way for a full-body orgasm.

o **Tantric Yoga**

Tantric yoga helps improve the nature of one's relationship and cherishes and imparts delicate exercise to accomplices. It is an easy-to-execute yoga routine for sex accomplices to build the progression of sex yielding energy. It additionally helps in standard practice for making your body resistible, with a decent body, personality, and soul both inside and outside the room.

o **Straightforward Yoga Movements**

This segment will enable you to get familiar with a couple of fundamental yoga represents that you can perform to improve your general wellbeing and stamina. In the following segment, you will learn about the diverse tantric activities you can, and your accomplices can perform together. This will help in expanding your closeness and solace level with each other.

o **The Head Lift**

Ensure that you are standing up straight for this. At that point tilt your head upward, what's more, tilt it in such a way, that string from the sky was pulling it upwards. Keep your mouth shut, and you should breathe in through your nose. When you are breathing in, ensure that you are moving your shoulder bones in reverse to appear that they are attempting to contact one another. It should feel like your feet are fixed to the ground. Loosen up your position and afterward rehash this procedure.

o **The Cobra Postures**

You can rest on the floor or a yoga tangle. Presently stretch out your body to make sure that your stomach is contacting the floor. At that point place your hands under your bears with the goal that your elbows are set at the back. Lift your chest off the floor also, tilt your head with the goal that it would seem that a bend. Ensure that you are looking upwards. This posture should like a cobra that is going to strike. Loosen up your position and after that recurrent this procedure.

o **The Cat Postures**

When you are finished with the Cobra present, you should delicately bring down your head furthermore, gradually ascend on your knees. This should appear as though you are squatting, so stretch your spine the other way than what you did in the Cobra present.

o **The Resting Postures**

When you have completed the Cat present, you should expect the Cobra present. Stretch your arms outwards. Take in profoundly and unreservedly. Ensure that your temple is lying on the ground and that your chest is contacting your knees.

o **Tantric Exercises**

If you need to add some use to your routine with regards to Tantric sex, at that point, you can start rehearsing a couple of activities and breathing procedures that will help you in making your sexual experience far and away superior. Just as relaxing systems, these activities are most appropriate when finished with your accomplice, yet they should be possible on your own also. These activities and breathing systems have been referenced in this segment.

- **Shoulder Stand**

  Shoulder stands are useful for ladies for accepting the different Tantric stances effortlessly, yet on the other hand, men can rehearse them also. For playing out a basic shoulder represent, the individual should rest level on a tangle or even the floor with his/her legs extended straight and their hands resting close by. At that point, the individual will need to lift the legs at a 90-degree edge to achieve their upper-middle stay stuck to the floor. Their legs ought to be lifted somewhat higher than their lower back, and their hands ought to be put on their back for supporting this pose. Rehearsing this strategy will help in building up the truly necessary adaptability for accepting different Tantric sex positions.

- **Boat Posture**

  This posture is by and by supportive for ladies. The individual playing out this posture ought to sit with a straight back, and their legs ought to be loosened up. At that point, the individual should lift their legs at a 45-degree end and, after that, stretch their hands outwards with the goal that their fingers are pointing towards their feet. Attempt and keep up this posture for three minutes and after that, unwind. Rehash this posture multiple times.

○ **Three-Legged Pooch Posture**

This posture is useful for extending the hamstring muscles, and these are very regularly utilized in Tantric sex. For playing out, this represents, the individual must lie down on their stomach on a tangle while their hands are set on their sides. Your palms ought to be placed alongside the chest and bolster your feet with your toes. Lift your body in such a way that your toes maintain your body weight. This position ought to appear as though your body is making a triangle, with the floor framing the triangle's base. The correct leg should then be gradually lifted upwards. Lift your leg to the extent your body would allow. At that point, come back to a nonpartisan position and rehash the equivalent with the other leg.

○ **Extension Posture**

This is a representation that is appropriate for both genders. For playing out this procedure, you should rest on your back, and, after that, twist your legs in such a way so your knees are pointing upwards. Your feet ought to be set near your bum. The lower middle ought to be lifted, and your hands should lie on either side of your body for offering help. Rehash these multiple times.

CHAPTER 10:

Tantric Sex Positions

R ight now, you will find out about various Tantric sex positions and procedures that you can use for spicing up your sexual coexistence.

The Sidewinder

This position is animated from a similar name's yoga position, and this procedure takes into account deep entrance.

It likewise accommodates the couple to keep in touch. For playing out this method, the lady should rest on her side and support her chest area's heaviness with her hands' assistance.

She should lift one of her legs and place it on her darling's shoulder while the other portion is lying on the bed.

A variety of this equivalent position is that the man can rest behind the lady and enter his partner.

The Yab Yum

The Yab Yum position is viewed as probably the best situation for having tantric sex. It is a genuinely simple situation to perform, and it takes into consideration synchronous climaxes. This position helps in animating quite a few places. Likewise, the man's hands happen to be free right now, he can touch his darling's body however he sees fit, since the couple would confront one another, it takes into consideration enthusiastic kisses also. The man should sit leg over leg on the bed or some other agreeable surface and hold his back straight. The lady should straddle him and fold her legs over his lower back. It takes into account delayed here and there developments that can help the couple in accomplishing an all-around planned climax.

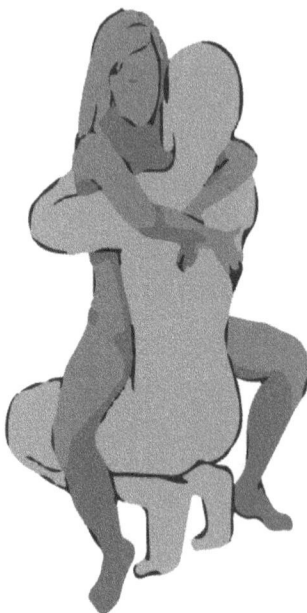

The Latch

This posture permits the man to get a decent see his sweetheart's face and the other way around.

This is an extremely attractive posture and aids in pleasuring both partners.

For playing out this procedure, the lady should be situated on a high stage like a table or even the kitchen counter. S

he will then need to recline and adjust her upper-middle and head with her hands' assistance by inclining onto her elbows.

The man should remain between her separated legs and enter her.

This represents that doesn't need to be limited to the room and is ideal for an off-the-cuff cavort.

The Butterfly

This method is accepted to allow both the partners to achieve a significant level of rapture and consider deep entrance. For playing out this system, the young lady should rest on the table so that her butt lies at the edge of the table. The man should help lift her lower back marginally off the table and afterward place both her legs over his shoulders. Her vagina would be free for him to infiltrate while remaining in the middle of her legs. Since her legs are shut together, this fixes the vaginal waterway and gives a tight fit. The man should enter her while her butt is in midair.

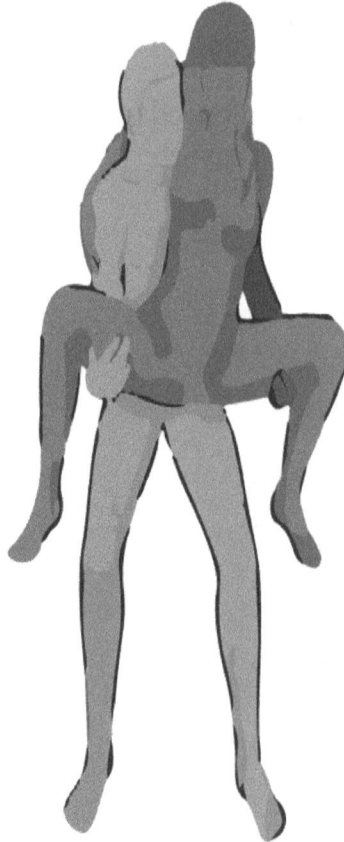

The Double Decker

This is an amazingly suggestive posture and will help in accomplishing a climax with no problem at all. The man will likewise be given a decent perspective on all the activity going on down there, and his hands will likewise have unlimited access to lay with his sweetheart's butt. This position is very enabling for ladies since they have all the control here. For playing out this system, the man should sit on the bed while his legs are collapsed under his body. The lady will then need to confront him and place her feet on either side of her darling while her feet are set level superficially to give her some help. When she has brought down herself onto his erect penis, she will just need to begin moving advances and reverse or even decide on a here and there movement. The man should kick back and have fun.

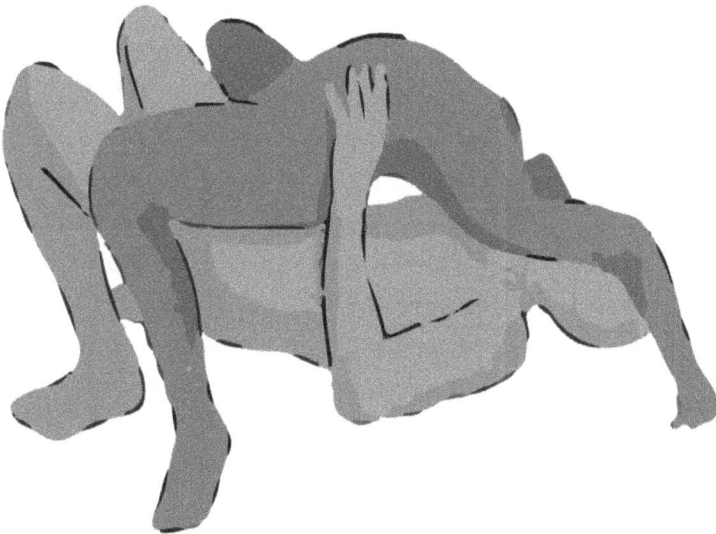

The Last Place Anyone Would Want to Be
This is an extraordinary posture since it permits both the gatherings to have a similar control measure and ooze a similar measure of pressure for having a great sexual encounter. People will have an equivalent balance right now. For playing out this represents, the man should sit on the bed and support his chest area with his knees. He will then need to move the lower portion of his legs in reverse and place them marginally separated. The lady will then need to expect a similar position. Yet, she will do as such while confronting ceaselessly from him and her run would be squeezing into his scrotum and her back against his chest. Her legs would be joined and afterward set in the space that is accessible between his legs and the man should enter her from behind. For this situation to be compelling, both the partners should remain as near to one another as could reasonably be expected.

Skiff
This position is a slight adjustment of the lady on top position. Right now, bodies should be situated so that both the partners will find a good pace great take a gander at one another's face while occupied with the demonstration. For playing out this, the man should sit down on a seat that can marginally twist in reverse. The lady will then need to put herself on his lap and place her legs on either side of the seat. The young lady should fire an allover development without anyone else. Her partner can help her by setting his hand under her bum and helping her move in an upwards and downwards way.

The Mermaid

This is a somewhat fluctuated adaptation of the butterfly, and it takes into consideration a more solace and better hold. Right now, a man can play with his darling's feet. Remember that feet are viewed as one of the most touchy and erogenous pieces of a lady's body. For playing out this method, the lady should expect a similar situation as she did in the butterfly, however, her butt ought to be propped with the assistance of a pad. Her legs should loosen up and ought to be at a 90-degree edge. The man should stand near the table and infiltrate her.

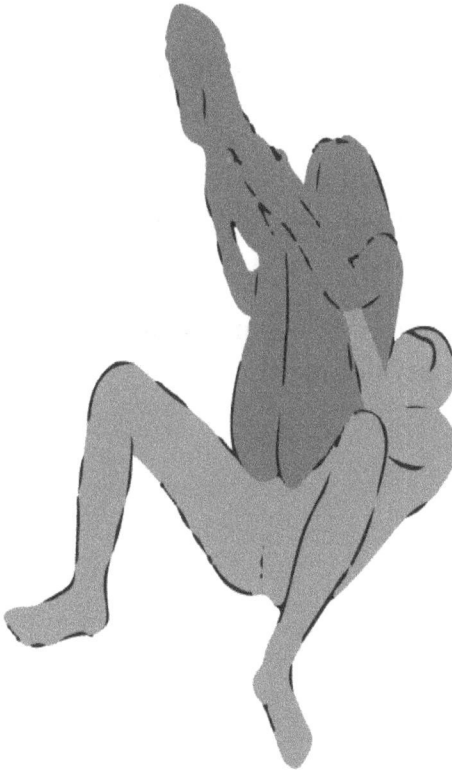

Tsunami

This posture is very agreeable, and it is a sensual treat.

This will knock your socks off.

This posture is a slight alteration of the exemplary minister style.

Right now, a lady should expect the job that a man, as a rule, does in the teaching style.

The man should rest level on his back for playing out this, and his arms should be put close by.

The lady should lie over him, and the man should embed his penis into her vagina.

The lady should loosen up her legs with the goal that they are resting on him. Her palms ought to be put on his lower arm for giving her some help.

The lady will then need to begin moving her pelvis in an upward and descending development.

Lap Dance

This is a great posture for a man to encounter his darling's body in the entirety of its magnificence. His hands will be allowed to meander around her body, and he can do what he needs. The lady will face away from him as she would have, had she been giving him a lap move. The man should sit down on a seat for playing out this represents, and his back should be kept straight. The lady will then sit on his lap and parity herself by setting her hands on his upper thighs or even his stomach. She will then need to lift herself gradually and place the backs of her calves and brings down herself onto his penis. Another variety of this would be that the lady should bring down herself onto his penis while confronting her darling. This will give him a serious decent perspective on her bosoms. He can choose to prod and play with them for whatever length of time that he satisfies.

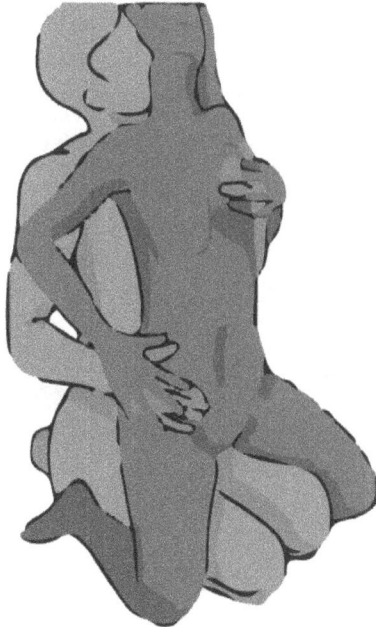

Pretzel

This is another representation that is satisfying to take a gander at and even simple to expect. This will cause the couple to feel incredibly attractive. For playing out this procedure, the couple should stop before one another. The man should move advances, and the lady will fold her arms over him. The lady will then lift herself and place her left leg by her darling's correct foot; her foot will confront downwards. The man will then need to put his left leg close to her correct foot. When taken a gander at a couple occupied with this posture, they look like a pretzel, an extremely provocative and mouth-watering pretzel.

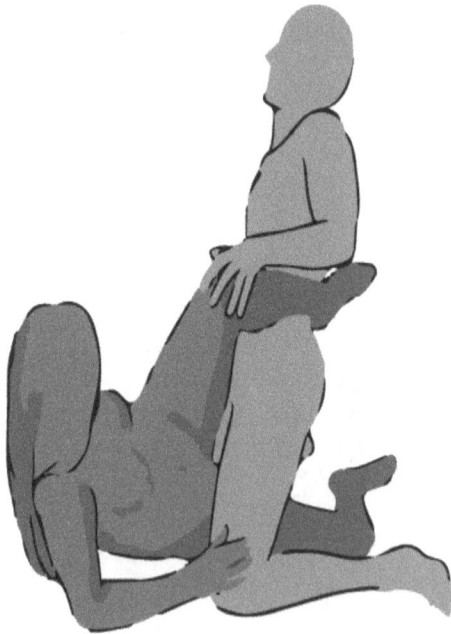

The Spread

This is an essential and amazingly hot position. This permits the lady to get incredible delight since it lets her stroke her sweetheart and permits him the entrance to joy her. For playing out this system, the lady should sit at the very edge of the couch or even the bed and spread her legs separated. The man will then need to remain in the middle of her legs and infiltrate her. She can draw nearer to him and kiss him while his hands have her full body entrance.

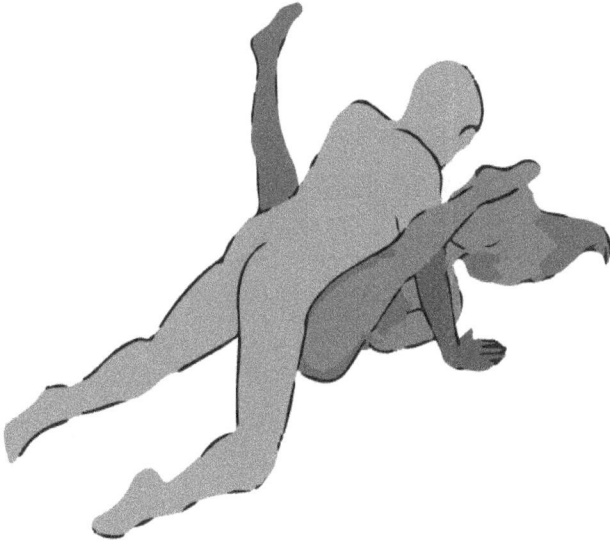

The Entwine

This posture looks intense and about difficult to copy, however, then it very well may be pleasurable if it's done appropriately. This posture is tastefully engaging.

For playing out this strategy, the couple should sit near one another and face each other.

The man should put his legs on either side of his partner.

The lady will then need to lift both of her legs and place them on either side of her sweetheart's sides, under his arms.

The man's upper arms will secure the lady's legs, and the lady will then need to lift her upper arms and place them over his elbows.

The man will then lift his legs and place them over her hands. This does sound very messy, isn't that right?

All the exertion that goes into it will merit your time and energy.

The G-force

This is maybe one of the most blazing tantric sex presents there is. This is the piece de opposition of all sex presents. The man has full oversight over his darling right now. Both the people included will get extraordinary delight from this posture. For playing out this position, the lady should rest on her back on the bed, and the man must bow by her legs. He will then gradually lift her middle off the bed so she's offsetting herself with her head and her shoulders put on the bed. The man can either extend her legs at a 90-degree edge or infiltrate her, or he can likewise pull them separated and place her feet just beneath his chest and enter her.

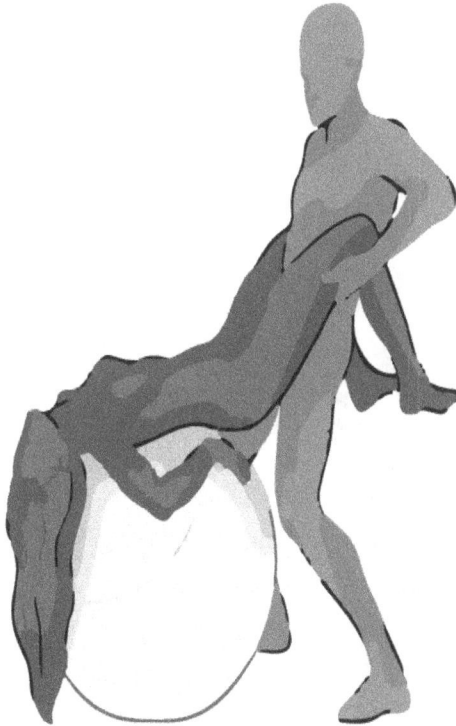

The Waterfall

Right now, a lady should put her hand on her sweetheart's penis and afterward let her fingertips brush his scrotum gradually and tenderly. It is a smart thought to use some ointment for making it progressively pleasurable. Her hands should be set on either side of his gonads, and afterward, she should gradually slide her hands up till they arrive at the touchy tip of his penis. When this is done, the lady should give the man some time to chill off, and he will then need to respond to the administration he got. The man needs to cup his sweetheart's vagina and touch all her delicate spots. He should slide his hands over her clitoris and her vaginal external lips.

The Snake

For this, the lady should gradually extend the pole of her sweetheart's penis with one of her hands and let the other hand follow little circles directly under the leader of the pole. This is like giving slow and delicate handwork.

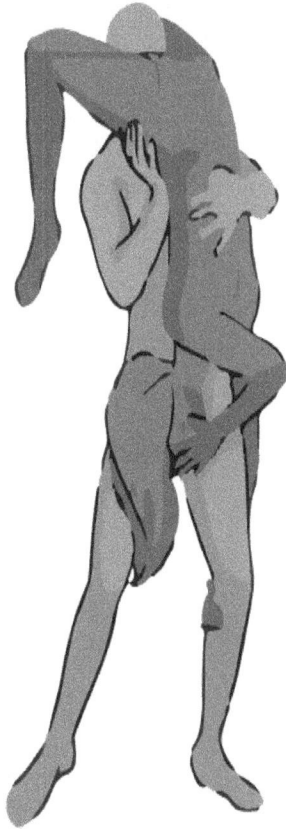

CHAPTER 11:

Multiple Orgasm

The orgasm has long been viewed as the peak of sexual excitement. It's a very powerful feeling of pleasure, which involves releasing accumulated erotic tension. While everybody's goal with sex is an orgasm, there isn't a lot known about it. During the last few centuries, theories about the orgasm have changed. For example, experts have only recently started talking about female orgasm. Many doctors in the 1970s claimed that it was perfectly normal for a woman not to experience an orgasm. Orgasms can be defined in several ways with different criteria. Medical professionals talk about physiological changes that happen within the body. Mental health professionals and psychologists talk about cognitive and emotional changes. There is not a single, overarching definition of the orgasm. Sex researchers have tried to define orgasms in models of sexual response. While the process for orgasm can differ between people, several basic physiological changes often occur in most incidences.

Master and Johnson's Four-Phase Model includes:

- Excitement

- Plateau

- Orgasm

- Resolution

Kaplan came up with his model, but he differs from most sexual response models because it includes desire. The majority of models don't include non-genital changes. It's important to understand, though, that not every sexual act is preceded by desire. Kaplan's three-stage model is:

- Desire

- Excitement

- Orgasm

Benefits of Orgasms

A 1997 cohort suggested that men's mortality risk was lowered when they experienced a high number of orgasms than in men who had fewer orgasms. There is also some research that suggests ejaculation can help to reduce the risk of prostate cancer. Researchers found that a man's prostate cancer risk was 20% lower in those who ejaculated at least 21 times a month than those who ejaculated only four to seven times a month.

There are a lot of hormones that are released during orgasm, which includes DHEA and oxytocin. Some studies suggest these hormones may help protect against heart disease and certain cancers. Oxytocin, as well as other endorphins that are released during the female and male orgasm, are also relaxants.

Types of Orgasm

Not surprisingly, since experts haven't reached a consensus regarding a definition of an orgasm, there are many different types of orgasms. Sigmund Freud stated that female orgasms as clitoral in immature and young, and vaginal in women with a healthy sexual response. In contrast to this, Betty Dodson has said that at least nine different orgasms are biased towards genital stimulation. We'll go over a few of those types.

- Tension orgasms – This is a common type of orgasm. It is created through direct stimulation, often when the muscles and body are tense.

- Relaxation orgasms – This orgasm comes from deep relaxation through sexual stimulation.

- Pressure orgasms – This orgasm comes from indirect stimulation of applied pressure. This is a type of self-stimulation that is common in young people.

- Multiple orgasms – These are a series of orgasms that happen over a short period.

- Blended or combination orgasms – These are a variety of orgasmic experiences that blend together.

There are a few orgasms that both Dodson and Freud discounted, but others believe they are real. For example:

- G-spot orgasms – This is an orgasm that is caused by the stimulation of an erotic zone in the vagina through penetrative intercourse, which feels very different from orgasms caused by other forms of stimulation.

- Fantasy orgasm – These are orgasms that result from mental stimulation.

The Female Orgasm
Men and women go through similar yet different physiological processes when experiencing an orgasm. Here we will talk about the process of the female orgasm following the Masters and Johnson four-phase model.

1.   **Excitement**

When a woman is psychologically or physically stimulated, the blood vessels in her genitals will dilate. This increased blood flow will make the vulva swell, and fluid will pass through the vaginal walls. This makes the vulva wet and swollen. Internally, the vagina expands at the top. Breathing and heart rate will quicken, and her blood pressure will rise. The blood vessel dilation can cause a woman to look flushed, especially on the chest and neck.

2.   **Plateau**

As the blood flows to the lower vagina area, it will reach a limit and turn firm. Breasts can also increase in size by 25% and increase the blood to the areola, making the nipples look less erect. The clitoris will then pull back against the pubic bone, making it look like it has disappeared.

3.   **Orgasm**

The genital muscles will experience rhythmic contractions that are about 0.8 seconds apart. For women, their orgasms last longer at about 13 to 51 seconds. Since women don't have a recovery period, they can continue to experience orgasms if stimulated again.

4.   **Resolution**

The body will slowly return to its previous state, reducing breathing, pulse rate, and swelling.

The Male Orgasm

1.   Excitement

When a man experiences psychological or physical stimulation, he gets an erection.

Blood flow increased in the corpora, which is the tissue that runs throughout the penis, which causes the penis to grow and become hard. The testicles will draw up as the scrotum tightens.

2.   Plateau

With the increased blood flow, the testicles and glans will increase in size. The buttock and thigh muscles will tense, the pulse quickens, blood pressure rises, and breathing increases.

3.   Orgasm

Semen, a mixture of 95% fluid and 5% sperm, is forced through the urethra by contractions in the pelvic floor, vas deferens, seminal vesicles, and prostate glands.

These contractions also cause the semen to be forced out of the penis, causing ejaculation. Orgasm for a man tends to last for ten to 30 seconds.

4.   Resolution

The man is now in the recovery phase, where he can't have any more orgasms.

This is what is called a refractory period, and how long it lasts varied between men. It could be a few minutes to a few days and tends to become longer the older the man becomes. At this point, the testicles and penis return to their original size. Their pulse and breathing will be fast.

Multiple Orgasms

People find the idea of multiple orgasms intriguing and for a good reason. It is perfectly normal to want to experience one right after the other and simply tapping out after the first. Here, we will discuss why the female body is designed to experience multiple orgasms, and strategies to make them more likely to happen.

Having multiple orgasms doesn't necessarily mean that you have another orgasm right after your first one without a moment's rest, but you can do that. Multiple orgasms simply mean that you have several orgasms during a single sexual encounter.

To experience multiple orgasms, will require some experimentation on your part. After you have your first, you will need to figure out what can make it happen again. If you find that your clitoris is so sensitive that you can't touch it, use the rest of your body. Try out different forms of stimulation. This could be playing with your breasts or getting your partner to kiss everything except the clitoris. The main point is to continue the arousal in whatever way works for you. Continue this for however long you want. You can always check back in with the clitoris to see if some of the sensitivity has gone away.

That being said, sometimes stimulating the sensitive clitoris could be the ticket. Some women say continuing to run the clitoris gives them the chance to embrace what seems like unbearable overstimulation, which can result in more orgasms. It all depends on what you can handle. If you like oversensitivity, then do it. If it hurts or can't see it creating a pleasurable feeling, don't continue touching it just to try and have more orgasms.

You can also use Kegal exercises to help extend your orgasms. As you reach your first orgasm, push your hand over your vulva and pulse it between orgasm contractions as you squeeze your thighs. Doing this can intensify and increase the orgasmic contraction and bring you into another orgasm.

You also need to make sure that you breathe during the entire experience. There are some people who will unconsciously hold their breath as the orgasm builds, but concentrating can help. When you reach or orgasm, breath purposefully, slowly, and deeply while contracting your pelvic floor muscles. This breathwork can lead to multiples for some people.

These tips are a great place to start but don't get upset if they don't work the first time. It takes practice and learning your body.

CHAPTER 12:

Tips to Improve Tantric Sex

More often than not, when an orgasm is achieved, it will be by one party or the other. It is fairly rare for both people to achieve orgasm at the same time. There may have been occurrences where this has happened for you and your partner. Still, it was likely not on purpose, and repeating it, if you tried, was probably quite difficult.

We will provide you with information on how you and your partner can work together so that you can orgasm together. If you have never experienced a mutual orgasm with your lover, it is something for the record books. Many couples have heard about this but have never experienced it. By gaining some information, you will likely be able to climax together and share an experience unlike any other.

Having an orgasm at the same time as your partner will truly deepen your connection. You will likely be more in love with them than ever before when you can experience something like this. When our body's orgasm, they release hormones; if this occurs simultaneously, it will help both of you become more in tune with the other. It cannot only enhance your sex life but also your relationship.

You want to keep in mind that it takes women longer to reach orgasm than it does men. By implementing extra foreplay, you can make it easier for your lady. Clitoral stimulation is a great way to help her achieve orgasm more easily. One way to provide extra sensation to her clitoris is for her to cross her legs while you are in just about any position. It will slow things down, which will make him last longer, and it will also allow his pelvis and member to stimulate the clitoris.

A big part of reaching orgasm together is to slow everything down. Men tend to reach orgasm when they have deep penetration and arrhythmic style of stimulation. If you notice he is getting close, the best thing you can do is limit his penetration level and slow everything down to a turtle's pace. The female will likely want to be the one in control of this as when he is close to orgasm, he may not think about it. Communication is also going to play a role, make sure your partner is letting you know if they're getting close. This will allow you to decide if you are close enough to make it to or if you need to slow things down and make the process longer.

Eye contact during intercourse is also critical. This is especially true if you are trying to orgasm together. When we can look into each other's eyes, it is a very intimate thing. It also gives off a very good set of nonverbal cues that allows your partner to understand when you are getting close to the climax. The fact that eye contact can be difficult to maintain, but with practice, it becomes easier. Taking the time to get comfortable looking into each other's eyes for long periods can make it easier for the two of you to orgasm together.

Allowing the woman to be in control is also advantageous. Because her orgasm is going to take longer, allowing her to be in control will let her set the pace so that you guys have a chance of orgasming together. The best positions to do this would-be one like cowgirl or her straddling him on a chair. The motion that works the best for her will be achieved in these types of positions. Additionally, they allow for easy clitoral stimulation. As we know, double stimulation for a female makes achieving orgasm a much simpler thing.

If simultaneous orgasm is the goal, you should never be afraid to stop. Simply stopping it while intercourse is still happening can be nearly impossible when we are close to climax. If you notice your partner is getting close, but you still need more time simply stop the activity. Spend some time kissing, cuddling, and caressing each other. This can help to calm things down but still, keep your partner aroused. After things have settled down and orgasm is no longer ready to happen, you can continue having sex. This tactic can be implemented at any point during your lovemaking sessions.

Something that may take a little practice but can be super helpful is when men learn to do Kegel muscle exercises. Sure, this is a thing that most women are already doing to make sure that they have strong pelvic floor muscles and that they feel tight during penetration. Men have the same muscles on their pelvic floor. When these muscles are strengthened, they can help him last longer. If your man is about to reach orgasm, have him perform an extended Kegel muscle exercise and take a few deep breaths. More often than not, this will help the urge to climax subside. Additionally, the more he practices this technique, the better it will work.

Speaking of Kegel muscles, they can also be utilized by the female. If a woman performs Kegel muscle tightening during intercourse, it can help her reach climax faster. It helps to build arousal because of the increased blood flow to the area that these exercises cause. The feeling of this can also be quite stimulating for the man. The bottom line is that everyone should be doing Kegel muscle exercises inside and outside the bedroom. They are a good variety of benefits to doing so.

The motions that you use during intercourse will also play a major role. Many men find that the in and out motion gets them and allows them to reach climax easily. So, by switching up the motion so that it is rocking or grinding rather than thrusting in and out, you can make him last a lot longer, giving the female more time for her orgasm to build up. Rocking motions are fantastic as they also allow for clitoral stimulation regardless of the position you may be in. So, even if your hands aren't free, get to rocking and realize how quickly you can achieve orgasm together.

Don't be afraid to provide yourself with extra stimulation if you need to achieve orgasm. This goes for the man or the woman. Clitoral stimulation is always going to help a woman achieve orgasm more quickly but paying attention to other erogenous zones of the body can also be beneficial. Maybe your man has an extremely sensitive spot on his shoulder, or he is into anal stimulation by paying attention to these areas you can get your partner going. Conversations and paying attention to each other can help you both understand the best ways to ensure that simultaneous orgasms can happen from time to time.

Another great thing to keep in mind if you are trying to orgasm together is that adding pressure to the base of a man's penis can help stop his orgasm in its tracks. Whether his female counterpart does it or he does it himself, trying to stop an orgasm can be made a bit easier by using this tactic. When you are truly in the moment, it can be a bit hard to remember, but it'll be worth the time to implement this.

You must understand that if you are going to have a simultaneous orgasm with your partner, it will not be during a one-night stand. You need to know the person and be able to read their cues to make it happen. When you understand their physical responses and how their body reacts before orgasm, it provides you with the information you need to stop or keep going. Mutual orgasms are a thing of trial and error. It is likely you will need to keep at it to make it happen and tweak things so that each time you get closer to it happening.

There is no rush in making this type of thing happen. It just takes practice and communication. Discussing your sex session after it happens and figuring out what you can do to prolong the session to the point of you climaxing together is advantageous. Don't get stressed out if you can't make it happen right away, instead enjoy the time you get to spend with your partner trying.

Another trick that can help you achieve a simultaneous orgasm is almost as good as eye contact. We're talking about synchronizing your breathing. Synchronizing your breath with another person does take a bit of time. The best way to do it is in a position where the female's back is against the male's chest. This will allow her to feel him breathe and make her breathing pattern the same. It is amazing how intimate it is when you start to breathe in the same rhythm as your partner. By maintaining this matched breath achieving mutual orgasm is significantly easier.

Sometimes it's hard for people to find the words they want while in the throes of passion. You can come up with a fun code for you and your partner so that there is a mutual understanding of how close to climax each of you is. You can do this with simple things like squeezing each other's hands or how you touch each other can change. It can be quite fun coming up with the system, so the other one knows if you are only 50% of the way there or if you are right around the corner from achieving orgasm.

All in all, you need to remember that intercourse with your partner is supposed to be fun. It should not be a stressful situation. Sure, achieving mutual orgasm is something that everyone wants to experience, but it does take some time and practice. Stay calm and know eventually you guys will be able to get there together.

Once you have been able to climax together, it is likely that you are going to want to do it again. Trying the same tactics may be the best avenue to ensure that you can repeat the process. However, spicing things up and doing things differently each time can also be advantageous. It keeps both parties on their toes and can make having sex more fun in the long run.

Conclusion

Tantric sex positions' is an excellent short fictional story that will allow you to see the tantric sex practice from various perspectives. The tantric sex practice does not need any fabrication to make it appear valid. It is reasonable, as it is stated. It can show you how to feel the energy in the body before any actual sexy action happens.

The Tantric sex practice is about developing the interconnectedness of the universe. It creates a robust and energetic connection.

Tantric sex helps in learning how to feel the energy in the body before it acts. This is part of intelligent sexual development.

Tantric sex practice does not require any physical intercourse action. All Tantric sex practices are based on the inner story and not on the action happening externally. Tantric sex teaches people about the fullness of the sexual pleasure experienced by connecting the sexual organs in a certain way.

The Tantric sex practice in itself does not need an orgasm to happen as sometimes people think. This is not a cock and ball or pussy and cock kind of act. This does not require penetration. Sexual organs are not present in Tantric sex practices, but they are utilized.

An orgasm can be experienced by practicing Tantric sex practice if practicing in different positions and comfortable and relaxed enough.

When practicing Tantric sex in conjunction with pure sexual practices, an orgasm can be experienced.

Some people think that Tantric Sex is an Ejaculation kind of sex, but this is not true as the orgasms taken after Tantric sex practice are not meant for cock and balls ejaculation. Still, they are meant for experiencing and understanding the body.

Some involuntary actions often accompany the non-ejaculatory orgasms that occur with the Tantric sex practice. This might happen only once in a lifetime, during the Tantric sex practice.

Tantric sex can be practiced with a partner and without a partner. It is based on internal energies and not on the physical act happening externally.

The tantric process is devoted to discovering energy at its highest level through the various practices of yoga, meditation, and other disciplines. The methods are then used to develop the strength and help move it from the lower chakras to the highest chakra, the crown chakra, in the head's back.

Practicing tantric sex is also an exercise in creating a beautiful energy flow. It is an art form. We are living, breathing, organic sculptures... dynamic, vital, sensuous. Sex in itself is an art form. The following scenarios are meant to be simply suggestions — ways to bring tantric sex into your intimate life. They do not prescribe any specific actions or techniques but simply provide some starting points. Just follow the natural direction of your instincts. You are the artist, the breath, the beauty.

As you practice and learn the simplicity of this approach, you may be astounded by how it helps you and your partner experience a level of intimacy that you never thought was possible. And I am not just talking about the emotional and spiritual side of sex. I am talking about all the aspects of sexual pleasure.

You will notice that tantric sex doesn't necessarily require penetration, or orgasm, or ejaculation. Ejaculation can often hinder the fullness of sexual experience. If you are engaged in tantric sex, then you can develop many different tantric sex practices without the need for "coming."

Yet you can easily add those practices as you progress. And if they feel right, simply intensify them. How you experience sex depends on several factors that can change over time. How's your health? How easily can you relax? How much sexual experience do you have? How available is your partner? How much time do you have?

But whatever those variables, tantric sex can be a most profound and intimate experience, one that requires nothing more than you and your partner, your bodies, your breath, your consciousness, and each other.

KAMA SUTRA SEX POSITIONS GUIDE:

LEARN HOW TO SPICE UP YOUR COUPLE LIFE. FROM INTIMACY TO TECHNIQUES AND SEX GAMES, EVERYTHING YOU NEED TO ADD INTEREST TO YOUR RELATIONSHIP.

Table Of Contents

INTRODUCTION

I f you are reading this book, it is likely that you and your partner are looking for some hot ways to spice up your sex life. Rest assured, there are millions of couples, just like you, who are curious about how to improve their bedroom experiences and how they can share a more intimate relationship with each other.

We decided that the incredible gift of the Kama Sutra should be accessible to the common, everyday person that could use it for the benefit of their lives. Everyone deserves to have knowledge that will enhance their lives.

If you are relatively new to sex and you are looking for information, tips, and sex positions, this book will give you everything you need and more.

Read this book with an open mind and a willingness to learn. You will gain lots of new information in these pages, and it may seem overwhelming at first. The good news is, you can always flip back to any section and read it again if you forget some of the details.

There is much more to the Kama Sutra than just sex positions, and this book is aimed at teaching you everything it has to offer. It is about how to connect with a person, how to pleasure them, and even how to make them your spouse.

This book will give you the tools you need to fulfill your sexual fantasies and desires along with a bunch of extra, historical information to share with your lover – maybe even practice?

Kama Sutra will teach you how to find pleasure in pleasuring someone else, and how to find pleasure through a series of locations on the body that are easily overlooked, especially during foreplay.

This book will give you insight on the practices of Kama Sutra and what is expected of the man and the woman in the relationship and the bedroom. This book will also make you aware of the general guidelines which male and females follow when attempting to pursue one another.

This book is geared towards couples, and has advice on moves and techniques that can enhance the intimacy and deepen the romance between lovers. Every single move or tip in this book will either assist in developing the intimate bonds between you two, or encourage you to have total trust in your partner while you are in a vulnerable state.

It is important to read this book together as a couple, as it can help encourage open lined of communication in the bedroom. This area of communication is just as important as elsewhere, as it helps us convey what we want, and what we don't want. Many people don't realize that we tend to evolve in our sexual desires the same way as we evolve and grow elsewhere in life.

As you explore this modern version of the Kama Sutra, be sure to take note on what you'd like to try, and then give it a shot. There is no right or wrong way to use this guide, simply do whatever feels right for the two of you. The most important thing is to let loose and have fun!

So, relax is a warm place with a warm beverage or your favorite wine or relaxation libation and join us for the secrets of the Kama Sutra and enhance you life!

CHAPTER 1:

WHAT IS KAMA SUTRA

What is the Kama Sutra and its Myths Busted!

The Kama Sutra is more than just a sex guide, it's a philosophy that has gone back a thousand years and is still kicking. But because of the Eastern mystique, there have been some myths hanging around that have probably stopped people from wanting to read it.

Here, we are going to do something that is rarely done in books like this and that is bust the myths so you have a clear view going into these chapters.

First a Short History:

The Kama Sutra was written between 400B.C and 200 A.D. The authors name was Vatsyayana. He was a Hindu philosopher who actually wrote it as a guide to having a healthy sex and family life.

His very simple and profound philosophy stated that if you had a healthy sex life, you had a healthy mind and healthy lifestyle for life and would most probably live longer.

The creator of the Kama Sutra views love making and sex as a work of art. The Kama Sutra is a guide that also gives us a guide to how to get a wife, how to have sex and how to be attractive to the opposite sex. The Kama Sutra is so much more than the public who have heard of it know.

Myths Busted!

Myth One:
The Kama Sutra is a book of nothing more than sex positions.

The Kama Sutra is more a book of sexual science. It is one of those books with information that is never outdated. Why? Because it's not dogma. There is also another reason which is that people as a whole do not change. Sure we have technology and we advance intelligently over the years but people do not change. Sex is a part of life and always will be regardless of how we advance. So, this book could be buried in a time capsule and dug up a thousand years from now and will still hold the same value to the people that read it.

Myth Two:
The Kama Sutra is outdated

As it said in myth one, this book and it's philosophy can not be at all outdated. This is because this is a science that is related to the depths of man that is unchanging. There is a crazy notion that if there is something that is not associated with technology and was written by an ancient person in an ancient time that they are irrelevant. This is a crazy notion.

Myth Three:
The Kama Sutra only gives you physical techniques for better love making

This is only partly true. Though the book does cover the ins and outs of love making it also covers something much greater. It covers life in general and how releasing your sexual energy can cause you to have great health and well-being, make better decisions and have the best personal relationships. That's 10 X more valuable than just sex positions.

Myth Four:
The Kama Sutra is only for couples and only for those who want to put more spice into a dead sex life.

This could not be farther than the truth. Sure, the Kama Sutra will cover the best ways to spice up a dead sex life for sure but it also covers time you spend with a casual lover, spiritual partner and by yourself. Masturbation is a great part of the Kama Sutra because that is a fabulous way to release your sexual energy.

Today's Kama Sutra

Two thousand years after it was first introduced, the Kama Sutra is not only relevant, it has manifested itself in every from of art, entertainment and education.

During the middle ages, courtiers of the Muslim sultans that dominated India treated the "treatise on love" as nothing more than a sex manual, something to provide fantasies to their masters.

By the time the 1980's came around, the only thing had had changed was its circulation. The art books showcasing only the positions (and not the message) of the Kama Sutra reached Western culture. The Internet gave it even more popularity, but only as semi-pornographic material.

Various catalogs of the sexual positions were published, consisting of positions that weren't even included in the Kama Sutra. Not only had the message been stricken from these books, they presented a paint-by-numbers method of how to reinvigorate a couple's sex life. The positions were deemed pornographic, immoral and fodder for people of low standards.

Throughout the 1990's, a slow reemergence of the first publication began, and a society that long for sexual equality as well as sexual liberation began to embrace the meaning and intent of the Kama Sutra's positions.

The evolution of the Kama Sutra's reputation is most evident in today's entertainment. The ancient Indian text has permeated into movies and television shows on both sides of the globe, such as Sex and The City (US, 2000) and Kama Sutra: Tale of Love (1996, India/UK).

The Kama Sutra has inspired a wild range of artwork. From delicate paintings, to crude diagrams of the sexual positions to educate, to cartoon style interpretations to amuse, to erotic photo graphs to titillate, it would seem for every one of the original positions, there are hundreds of ways in which they've been depicted.

The publishing industry continues to give birth to new translations and interpretations of the Kama Sutra. There are also many novels and self-help books for couples that cater to beginners, experts and those with idle curiosity. Many of these manifestations of the Kama Sutra adhere to the books message of emotional and sensual connected-ness, but there are, of course, books that reduce the ancient tome as nothing more than kinky positions that can spice up any sexual encounter.

In an effort to educate the masses, seminars, workshops, magazine articles, websites and even blogs have committed to de-mystifying the Kama Sutra. Unfortunately, in attempt to make the material more accessible if not relatable, many of these formats focus on the thrill of trying the positions with little mention of intimacy. And when intimacy is encouraged, it's often done in the form of suggesting candles, perfumes and oils.

Perhaps by delving into the emotional work that the Kama Sutra entails, authors and moderators fear they may lose a large part of their audience. After all, in today's society, becoming emotionally naked sounds more like therapy than the beginning of an exploration into one's sexuality.

Ironically, modern culture has had only moderate success in getting the meaning of the positions to the masses, and yet it often gets confused with Tantra, which has a much stronger spiritual component than the Kama Sutra.

Kama Sutra Facts

Kama Sutra teaches many aspects of the sexual act.
There are four sections of one chapter of the Kama Sutra that deal with foreplay, after play, sexual congress and sexual preparation.

The Kama Sutra makes you more attractive
This is the part that teaches you the most valuable part you need in life to make your love life very successful. There is a magic when you learn what the other person's needs are this is a real connection which is the reason, they are attracted to you.

This also tells you how to set the mood and how to groom yourself to be ready for your encounter. It also tells you how to use sensual touches and techniques that you'll find in the Kama Sutra.

Benefits of Kama Sutra and Sex

Kama Sutra will bring you closer together.
This is all about experimentation here which Is a wild and wonderful thing. It states that if both partners take a sense of humor about it and laugh it off together when a position goes wrong or needs practice then you get closer.

The Kama Sutra teaches you the art of fellatio and cunnilingus

Most people have a way of approaching oral sex which is what is described above in the subtitle, in the same old way. This is a common thing and a lot of times, it's taken as a job with skills that are not that good because face it, most of us have no one to teach us and furthermore, the only role model they have is porn which is fantasy at best.

Kama Sutra makes you so much more confident

Being a great lover and partner and seeing the look on your partner's face will give you a very big confidence boost. When you're more confident doing one of the most nerve-wracking things and the thing that makes you the most vulnerable because you are naked, then, you can do anything.

Kama Sutra values empowering women

Despite all what our modern-day society keeps preaching about women and sexuality, Kama Sutra has a different view on this subject matter. Kama Sutra suggests that a woman needs to study the different forms of sex before she gets married. When a woman understands the different forms of sex, she would be a better mate and would be more desirable by her man. So, the Kama Sutra encouraging women and empowering them is one of the biggest benefits you stand to gain from the book.

Kama Sutra makes a clear classification of a man's penis

Also, the Kama Sutra made mention of the size of a man's penis and that it matters when choosing a mate. There are three types of man penis by Kama Sutra – the bull, horse, and hare. Kama Sutra also made mention of different sizes of woman's vagina, and that a perfect match of the vagina size and penis sizes would result in a good sexual experience.

Kama Sutra also emphasizes on living a healthy life and well-balanced one

Kama Sutra is also a book that talks about tips on how to live a healthy life. The Kama Sutra encourages that a man and a woman should embrace cleanliness which would, in turn, boost their health. A man, for instance, should shave his beard on a regular basis, and take his bath and eat healthily, and the same applies to a woman too. She should bread her hair and shave as well. Couples could also try mutual grooming.

Kama Sutra talks about enticing and approaching women

The Kama Sutra also talks about interesting tips a man can use to entice and approaching a woman. This tip helps men to know how to touch and caress a woman in other to express their desire when they want to have sex. When a man knows these various tips and how to use them, he will find it easier to get his message over to the woman. The tips of how to entice and approach a woman further move on to touching and embracing.

Kama Sutra talks about eight different types of embrace

There are different types of embrace from the Kama Sutra. It further tells us that there are up to eight different types of embrace which can be used for different purposes. Because of Kama Sutra teaching, we now know how to apply the various types of embrace. And on applying the right type of embrace at the right moment would set the right mood in motion. So, rather than keeping all your emotions inside, you can now use the various teaching from Kama Sutra about embrace to seduce and lure your lover into that perfect love zone.

Kama Sutra teaches about kissing

There are different forms of kissing too. Kama Sutra also teaches that a woman should feel too shy about a kiss. We all know that a man in most cases is the ones that initiate the kiss, but a woman should not feel shy to be the one to start the kiss first. There are also different types of kiss that partner can use to deeply connect with each other at particular points in your relationship. Like a type of kissing couples can engage in when walking on a lonely street. There are also different types of kiss that lovers can engage in when they want to make love.

Kama Sutra is divided into a set of 64 acts

Contrary to the belief that the Kama Sutra doesn't have a list of sex position howbeit lovemaking that includes penetration is divided into 64 acts. This acts explains the different ways couples can have sex to enjoy the maximum pleasure from sex. To have the best sex, you have to combine it with stimulating desire, and engaging in an embrace, caressing, kissing, biting, slapping, moans, oral sex, and everything in-between.

Kama Sutra recommends that your scratch your partner

There are different types of scratch you can have with your partner. With this knowledge Kama Sutra provide us, we can add a twist to lovemaking without loved ones. Moreover, leaving scratch marks on your lover's body can help keep the fire burning for each other even when your lover is not close to you.

Kama Sutra recommends that your woman lover should reach orgasm first

When making love with our loved once, Kama Sutra suggests that the woman should be the first to have an orgasm. This point is valid because of the extreme exhaustion a man feels after having an orgasm, whereby he wouldn't be able to proceed with sex at least not immediately. So, in other to have great sex, the woman should be the first to have an orgasm before the man allows himself to have an orgasm.

Kama Sutra also talks about a woman's sex as being more than just sex penetrations

In Kama Sutra, there is more to sex than penetration for a woman. To a woman, the whole act is sensual, but to a man reaches orgasm at the end of the intercourse. Most men think that making a woman have an orgasm is their ultimate act, but a woman needs both sexual and physiological pleasure to be able to satisfy her urge. Thanks to Kama Sutra, many men who were getting this concept wrong have been able to make adjustments.

Philosophy of the Kama Sutra

Looking at ancient Hindu texts, we know that the four virtues were commonly discussed and written at length about. Many of the texts focused on the two important virtues of Dharma (morality), and Athra (prosperity), while few really delved into the importance of Kama (pleasure). Vatsyayana meditated upon this reality and came to the conclusion that Kama was just as important as all of the other virtues, and so it was only proper to have a guide written solely about how to obtain Kama.

The four virtues can be looked at more as goals that each person much work towards within their lifetime in order to lead a complete and fulfilled life. Within the Kama Sutra, there are many references to the other virtues as they are all tied together and must be achieved in order to succeed. One cannot simply focus on the physical pleasures and ignore the need for morality or prosperity, so you may notice throughout that sex and morality are often combined, as well as sex and finding a partner that brings about monetary prosperity.

To understand the philosophy behind the Kama Sutra, it is vital that you understand what it was intended to be. The sex acts that are described throughout are little more than theatrics, with an emphasis on outrageous and yoga-inspired poses. The goal was unlikely to be used as a literal manual, but instead to be used as a way to understand both society and the individual. A vast majority of the book is taken up by discussing how men and women interact within society, both as a whole and simply with each other. It can be seen as almost a screenplay, taking us on a journey of love within ancient Indian times. There is talk of love, intimacy, and mundane tasks such as bathing and grooming. The Kama Sutra is a manual on all aspects of pleasure, both in the sexual sense and in the day to day realm.

Kama is so often seen as something that is less important than other aspects of human pursuit. We are told to work hard, earn money, find a spouse, have children, and live a moral and righteous life. But rarely are advised on how to let loose and enjoy ourselves, or how important of a role sex plays in the human experience. The Kama Sutra is the bridge over that gap, intended to lift up the importance of pleasure and sex, and place it in as high of regard as all the other aspects we are expected to work towards.

Some have questioned whether or not the Kama Sutra really is a female positive as it may appear, but if you approach it from the idea of the times, then it can actually be seen as more of a feminist work of art than the surface would suggest.

There is an obvious sexual freedom that is discussed within, one in which even our current societal viewpoint doesn't always acknowledge. Try bringing up the topic of female masturbation and see the sudden puritanical viewpoint that many people rush to. Movies are quick to showcase men in a sexual manner, but female sexuality is much more often subdued or removed completely from the narrative. To have a book that explores the different facets of a woman's sexuality is unique both historically as well as in the current climate. Given that the Kama Sutra talks almost nothing of procreation, it truly highlights the idea that this is a guide for pleasure and nothing more. So, by its own very nature, it is also a book dedicated to a woman's pleasure, both by herself and that which is given to her by her partner. Beyond just sex, the Kama Sutra also discusses how to treat a woman properly so that she is nurtured and cared for in all aspects of life. It discusses showering her with affection and gifts and giving her absolute power when it comes to the home's finances.

From a philosophical standpoint, the Kama Sutra opens our minds to the needs of both men and women, and it does a good job of including women in the discussion, especially for the times. Not only does it take a more liberal and open-minded approach to women, but that same approach is extended to homosexuality and bisexuality as well. There are many references and discussions about men sleeping with men, and women pleasuring other women, as well as advice on having threesomes and even orgies. Whatever the sexual desire is of the individual is both encouraged and celebrated, and there is no judgment cast upon those who may differ from what is considered the norm.

The Kama Sutra makes us think by challenging our conceptions and internalized beliefs when it comes to sex. Whether it is something we partake in or not, it opens our eyes to the different forms of relationships that can exist both romantically and sexually and offers up advice on how to succeed in achieving absolute pleasure. It removes the idea that sex should be for procreating and instead emphasizes the pleasure that can be found within a sexual encounter. On a deeper level, it challenges the notion that physical pleasure should take a backseat to otherworldly pursuits, and that pleasure is just as important in life as everything else. For a life without pleasure, it isn't truly a life worth living at all.

What Does it Teach Us?

The Kama Sutra teaches us many things, from how to take care of ourselves, to how to take care of our partner. Everything begins with you, and how you groom yourself and carry yourself in this world. It is an extremely practical guide, that mixes real-world advice with philosophical ideas and concepts. It is meant to make us sit back and think about why we do what we do, and how we can live a better life overall. But all of that begins with the individual person.

Even if we only look at the sexual aspect of the Kama Sutra, we can see exactly what the author is attempting to teach us about physical pleasure. None of us would exist without sex, so why do we diminish its role in our lives? The pleasure of the senses is literally necessary for life, so why not enjoy that and learn how to act upon those desires in both a free and moral way.

Beyond the sexual nature of the Kama Sutra, it also is a guide that teaches us how to live a good life in general. It goes in-depth on topics such as the arts, music, and literature, as well as how to be a good husband or wife. It discusses financial matters, matters of the home, and even how to properly select a spouse that is balanced with you. It goes into great detail about how you should bathe and groom yourself, where you can meet people, and how to enjoy your day and please your spouse.

From a philosophical viewpoint, it teaches us that both men and women should engage in sensual pleasures, and that sex is not just for men to get off with. Unlike many historical texts that downplay a woman's sexual desires, the Kama Sutra takes a deep look at what a woman's sexual nature is and how to properly satisfy it both before sex as well as during. That isn't to say, however, that the Kama Sutra is an extremely liberal book or that it holds men and women in the same regard. It is written during a time of caste systems and where women's role in a marriage was not as high as that of the man. Men were still considered the head of the household, and much of what is described revolves around a man pursuing a woman. But, compared with other forms of literature, it does take a more liberal view of women's sexuality, as well as homosexual relationships, and the idea of having sex solely for pleasure and outside of marriage.

How to Use the Kama Sutra?

The Kama Sutra can be used in two ways, both as a practical guide as well as a philosophical work of art. Some may approach the Kama Sutra only as a guide to sex positions and this is perfectly acceptable as a large chunk of text is dedicated to this pursuit. However, to use the Kama Sutra fully, you must look at it as a whole and take into account both the historical significance as well as the idea that it may not be as practical as one may originally think.

Many of the sex acts described within the Kama Sutra are outside a normal person's ability and require a high degree of flexibility to perform. There are even positions within the book that are physically impossible unless the man has a very uniquely shaped lingam (penis). Later in this book, we will look at some of the positions that are possible, however, and break down how exactly you can do them and incorporate them into your personal sex life. In many ways, there are a number of similarities between the sex acts within this book and the practice of yoga. Through breathing as one with your partner, folding into different positions, and experiencing everything in unity you can achieve a higher sense of awareness and satisfaction. So, even if you are unable to achieve the positions as described, think of it more like a workout for the mind and body and attempt a sexier form of yoga.

Since the positions are not always practical, you should use the Kama Sutra more as a general guide for how to deepen your pleasure. This book has taken many of the important concepts and ideas and broken them down into practical tips and advice so that you can elevate your sex life and truly engage in a more pleasurable and sensual experience. Beyond just the sexual side of it all, the Kama Sutra should also be used as a guide on how to treat your partner both inside and outside of the bedroom. It can assist you in being more romantic and intimate, as well as teach you how to make sure your partner is satisfied completely within the relationship.

With a breakdown of different personalities and temperaments, the Kama Sutra also discusses how you can go about finding the right partner for you based on ancient concepts and ideas. While some of the information may seem absurd in the context of today's world, not everything should be taken as a literal word. Instead, it is important that you read the Kama Sutra as a concept more than a script, and that between the lines you see that even the most ancient of dating tips is still applicable today.

CHAPTER 2:

LOVE AND THE KAMA SUTRA

When it comes to love, there is much that can be said on how to obtain it, maintain it, and nourish it. While sex and love do not always go hand in hand, the Kama Sutra does emphasize the importance of love and goes to great lengths in order to detail exactly how a person can find love and then how they should go about ensuring that it lasts for a lifetime. Love begins with oneself, and only then can it be extended beyond that and onto someone else. That is why the Kama Sutra makes sure to include ways to enhance your own inner love and desire but focusing on self-care and self-adornment. The more you love yourself the more you can love others, and the more they can love you in return. If you are down on yourself, lack self-worth, or generally feel unlovable, then you will project that onto everyone that you come in contact with. You need to be able to present the best version of yourself possible, and always remember, there is nothing sexier in life than confidence!

Love is an extremely complex concept, and while we all may feel we understand what love is, if you ask 100 individuals to define love you will end up with 100 different responses. Love is defined as the feeling of attraction and desire that one feels towards another, but if you have ever been in love you will know that it extends far beyond that shallow explanation. Love and lust can often be confused with one another, since both play on attraction and desire, but the simplest way to break the two apart is to see love as something that is long-term, whereas lust oftentimes will fade or develop into love. When it comes to love, there are many factors that go into both falling in love, as well as staying in love with someone. Love is not easy, nor is it free from work, and in order to maintain a healthy, loving relationship you must be willing to sacrifice, compromise, and put in effort daily. Love is something that can grow and deepen with time, like a tree grows its roots down into the earth. What begins as only a small sapling can eventually turn into a mighty oak that even the worst of storms cannot damage. But how does one grow that tree of love? And how does one nurture it so that it is not cut down with time?

What the Kama Sutra Says About Love

The Kama Sutra discusses love in-depth and focuses heavily on marriages as the best type of union. With that said, however, it does acknowledge that not all sexual relations happen within the confines of marriage, and it does discuss the varying types of relationships that can occur.

One part of the Kama Sutra that is important to take note of, is the fact that the author makes sure to point out that love alone is not enough to sustain a relationship, nor is it enough to make a person happy within their life. While love is an important part of pleasure and being satisfied, it cannot be the only thing that you rely on in order to make you happy. If you pin all of your hopes and expectations onto one person, you are going to find yourself let down and dissatisfied, as one person cannot possibly meet all of your needs and desires. Instead, you should look at love as one piece of the puzzle that is fitted with other aspects in order to create a beautiful image.

From a historical perspective, the concept of monogamy was not as enforced as it is in today's society, and instead, there were many courtesans, or prostitutes, that were utilized without judgment. The Kama Sutra makes many notes towards courtesans, as their role in providing the ultimate sexual pleasure was very important even though it may not have involved love. Since this isn't as applicable in today's world, however, we can adapt these teachings as more of a personal guide on how to behave. The reason why courtesans were so desirable is because they were generous lovers who focused on their partner's pleasure and had qualities about that that made them engaging and entertaining. While you should never be something you are not just to please someone else, the idea of working on your own personality and qualities to enhance them and make yourself more interesting is certainly not a negative. We should all work towards building up who we are, being confident in ourselves, and feeling free enough to express our innermost desires.

Physical Attraction and Love

Although love requires much more than a simple physical attraction, the way a person looks is oftentimes the first thing that draws us to them. When you are looking to meet someone, and you know nothing about them as a person, you are going solely off of how they look to you. If someone is physically unattractive in your eyes, there is very little chance that you will want to pursue something intimate with them and thus the road to love is cut short.

The Kama Sutra acknowledges this and spends a lot of time discussing how to make yourself more physically desirable so that you can ultimately find love. We are in no way suggesting that your appearance is the only thing about you that matters, but we are saying that you should pamper and care for yourself in order to be the best version of yourself that you can be. From good hygiene practices to wearing your favorite sexy dress, making yourself look good will also make you feel good and that creates an energy that will draw someone to you.

How to Find a Spouse

One area that the Kama Sutra goes very in-depth, is how to go about finding a spouse for yourself. There are a number of different sections that discuss this matter, and each provides practical tips to assist you. Some of the advice given may not be as applicable in today's world, as the invention of the internet has changed the dating landscape significantly. Also, many of us date for pleasure and not always with the goal of marriage, so this may not apply to everyone who is reading it. However, marriage was an important aspect of life back when the Kama Sutra was written, so it should come as no surprise that much of the book is written with married couples in mind. In the Kama Sutra, discussion about marriage begins with finding someone within the same caste as you, and nowadays this is not nearly as relevant. In modern times we avoid breaking people down into different caste systems, but there is some truth with regards to finding someone of a similar background. You want to ensure that you and your partner have similar beliefs and morals, as individuals who are too strongly opposed to the others' ideas may not work out in the long-term. This is especially important when it comes to key points, such as:

- Do you and your partner both want children?

- How do plan on raising those children?

- Are you devout in your religious beliefs?

- What are the ideas of gender roles within a marriage?

- Are your political beliefs similar?

- How you feel towards alcohol and drugs?

- Are your sex drives similar?

- Do you both want to get married?

- How do you approach financial matters?

- What do you expect from a partner?

- Where do you see yourself living?

- What are your main goals in life?

While a difference in opinion can be healthy and is even encouraged, if you differ on vital points then you are doomed to fail. If one of you dreams of being a parent, but the other is absolutely against having children, there will eventually be resentment between you as one partner will feel that a core desire is not being met. With regards to the Kama Sutra, the majority of the text on marriage discusses how a man should go about finding a wife and what he should look for in the woman that he marries. There is also a lot of discussion regarding marriages in which the man has multiple wives, and the role each wife should take in the relationship. This information is not as applicable today, so we have opted to leave it out of this chapter. But in order to properly cover everything that exists within the Kama Sutra, it is still worth mentioning that it exists. How one seeks out a wife is not the only thing that is discussed, and its fact the Kama Sutra goes into great detail regarding how a man should then pursue a woman and win her over. The Kama Sutra mentions the following in terms of what a man should avoid when looking for a wife:

- A man should not marry a woman who is asleep or crying

- He should not try and marry a woman who is already married

- He should avoid someone with a bad sounding name, or whose name ends in the letter R or L

- A man should not marry a woman who is disfigured, has crooked thighs, or is bald

- He should seek to marry a virgin who has reached puberty

- A man should not marry his friend or his sister

What we can take away from the above list is that times certainly have changed, and many of what is listed seems both childish and absurd by today's standards. However, some points, such as not marrying someone who is asleep or who is crying, are still very much valid and should be respected and adhered to! So, what should an ideal bride be?

- She should be beautiful to look upon

- She should come from a good family

- Her age should be three years or younger than the man

- She should be wealthy

- Her body should be in good health and have lucky marks on it

- She should not have been married previously

- Most importantly, she should be the one that the man loves

Now, that last point may seem contradictory to the others, for what if the man falls in love with a woman that is bald? Or a woman that is not three years younger than himself? Well, it is said in the Kama Sutra that above all else, the only that thing that will bring true happiness and prosperity is marrying someone that you are attached to and to whom you feel love. Without love, there is no reason to marry, and this is something we can attest to even today.

There are different types of marriages discussed within the Kama Sutra, but the main type is what is called Gandharva marriage. This is the type of marriage when two people are equally attracted to one another, and without any interference from others consent to be married. There are no rituals or family involved, and instead is private between the two who are to be wed. While this was seen as not socially correct, it is the type of marriage that is brought about due solely to love, and this is one of the highest forms of marriage attainable.

What we can take from the Kama Sutra in terms of marriage is that love should be the basis for a successful marriage. Regardless of what your spouse looks like, or what family they are born into, if you love the person you should seek them out and create that relationship with them. Looks will eventually fade, and social status can change, but what should be everlasting is the love you have for one another. As long as you have that, the marriage is starting out on the right foot.

CHAPTER 3:

SEDUCTION

L ife is a broad combination of factors that add up to a whole. All these factors don't exist in a vacuum. The universe, being a dynamic engine consisting of apparently opposite tensions and almost limitless variety, is the model of life itself. This can serve as the model of your lives together. Life's variety can't be segmented off and boxed into categories that isolate one of its features from all the others. The bits and pieces of our lives are not bits and pieces at all – they're dynamically interconnected, just as the universe itself is and as we all are with one another. Your romantic relationship, therefore, is designed to be the exemplar of a greater reality; a microcosm of reality itself.

Becoming divine in the flesh
Implicit in Kama Sutra is an invitation to all lovers to join in the cosmic dance. Whether we're aware or not, the joining of loving bodies in physical demonstrations of desire is a sacred act. Regardless of the nature of the act, to love physically is to participate in the divine dance. In making love with one another, we weave ourselves into the universe and come part of its integral whole. We help to hold it together.

If that sounds like a big responsibility, it's because you've never approached your sexuality from this standpoint before. When you actually undertake to do so, the whole thing becomes a lot less daunting. It just feels right. That's because it is.

Your sexuality and living it out in a wholesome, joyful way is part of the divine plan and an important component of cosmic harmony. When the energy that passes between two people is intense and incarnated through acts of physical intimacy, you draw closer to the divine without even understanding that's the case. The many moments of our live we spend in sexual congress, or in physical intimacy, are moments in which we lift the veil that conceals from us, in our everyday lives, the true nature of godhead.

We are part of it and in our sexuality, we are living out our most extravagantly divine natures. This is an awesome thought I'd like readers to make special note of. In fact, there's an exercise, I would encourage you all to try. Take off your clothes. Now, go look at yourself in a full-length mirror. Take the time to really look at yourself, to move your arms and legs, to smile at yourself and to examine the wonder of your beautiful, human body.

There may be some bumps, lumps, zig zags and ripples we look at and would prefer not to see. Every one of those presumed imperfections, though, is a wonderful and unique story about the incredibly individual nature of our bodies. We all have these unpredictable, ripply, lumpy, bumpy bodies. They share some common features. But our bodies are also specifically *us*. The human body is a tale of life and all it entails – the good, the bad, the challenging and the terrifying. Our bodies are like passports, stamped by our days and years with the experiences we've had, the adventures we've survived and the imprints of thousands of those who have come before us, making us who we are. We are incredibly complex beings and this is reflected in the wondrous human body.

Looking at your physical self and seeing yourself for what you are is a doorway to seeing others in the same, expansive and wonderstruck way. Your body isn't a crackerjack box. It's you. It's what people see and say, "There's thingamabob!" It's your calling card and your way of involving yourself in the day to day life of the world around you. Without it, you'd be a disembodied, amorphous Casper the Friendly Ghost, drifting about unnoticed (or perhaps scaring the living crap out of people). What I'm saying is simple – your body is what makes you human. All of it. Even the parts you don't particularly care for. Your body is your story.

The first and most important part of loving another person as they are, is loving yourself. When you can behold yourself nude and vulnerable, you'll be able to see your partner more compassionately, less judgmentally and more appreciatively. Now get ready to put that renewed vision of love to good use, as we explore the Kama Sutra's gifts to sexuality.

Your flesh is what the divine works with. God has no hands but ours. You are an instrument of the divine in the cosmos, working to hold together and uplift the harmonious interplay and balance of the universe. When the two become one, all is whole. When you love, the music of the spheres is heard, as the stuff of Creation is knit together again and sustained. Love is divine and making love as a co-creation of the universe, through every touch, every sigh and every movement of our bodies together, makes of us god's partners. Through our sexual natures, we come as close to the divine order in the cosmos as we may, as mere human beings, we become divine.

CHAPTER 4:

FOREPLAY

Foreplay

Foreplay is an incredibly important part of intercourse that many people don't pay enough attention to. When you've been together for a while, couples tend to only do the minimal work to get each other hot and bothered before they go at it.

If this sounds like you, spend a little extra time with foreplay. In fact, you can even span foreplay across a few days: giving each other oral or hand pleasure for a few days without ever allowing the other to orgasm, before finally diving into sex can be a wonderful experience for everyone involved.

The Best Kama Sutra Foreplay Techniques

Show each other you care

Remember that great sex starts and finishes in the mind. There are emotions that are needed to stir up the best in the relationship. The act of foreplay doesn't necessarily mean that there is a sexual act taking place at all. Foreplay really means whatever goes on prior to the act of intercourse.

That, for the Kama Sutra means to have a conversation about anything that relaxes the two of you. Go out into the fresh air, hold hands, build the mood and drink wine. Feed each other good food and be really in the now and with each other entirely.

Completely Embrace
There is something to be said for the good old-fashioned embrace! This does even more for the chemicals in your body. An embrace, whether it's with a human or with an animal, any warm blood loving embrace with another living thing does wonders for releasing the chemicals in the brain to the body.

Gentleman, use your teeth
According to the Kama Sutra, there are ways that you can use your teeth in any kissable area of a woman's body. The key is gentleness. You could even use your teeth to remove her clothes in part. Or, you could nibble lightly on the neck, the ear or her vaginal lips but remember to be gentle.

Let her be the advancer
The roles for men and women are clearly marked in the Kama Sutra but it is also very much encouraged that you allow her to take her sexual aggressions out on you with no issue. Let her act out as many fantasies as she wishes because this is the best thing to strengthen a relationship on the part of pleasing the female emotions.

Pleasuring Him
Men are largely stimulated by what they see, as well as physical experiences. In order to cater to these needs, we have comprised a list that primarily use your looks and touch to get him turned on. These tips are excellent ways to tease your man, and get him ready for what is yet to come. Of course, you can always add your own personal spin on these moves. After all, you know your man best!

Dress Up
This one might be a given. Wear a daringly short dress, some sexy lingerie, or dress up for your man's favorite sexual fantasy. Put some light makeup on, and let your hair hang down

naturally. Alternatively, you could wear pigtails or a pony tail for him to hold onto and ultimately mess up. You can also wear things that'll be able to stay on during sex, such as blindfolds, garter belts, stockings, or high heels. Jewelry can also enhance the visual experience. Go all out!

Wear Bold Lipstick

You might consider wearing a nice bold lipstick that compliments your skin tone. Typically, red is the color of choice for most, but you could also venture into a pink or magenta. Wear whatever you feel confident in. Be sure to leave lots of kiss marks in areas he can see later when he's cleaning up, such as on his lower tummy or his inner thighs.

Strip Tease

If you're dressed up for him, but plan on taking it all off, consider taking it off slowly. Dance around a little and give him a strip tease. Toss your clothes onto his lap while he sits back and watches you. You might even want to put on a sexy song to do this to, to enhance the mood.

Whisper in His Ear

When you're talking dirty to him, try whispering it in his ear. Use your breath to tickle the back of his neck, lick right behind his ear, or nibble on the lobe after you talk to him. These types of things can send shivers down his back and get him extremely turned on for you.

Get a Little Rough and Bossy

Men are almost always playing the dominant one in life. Give them a chance to know what it's like to be at your mercy by getting a little rough and bossy with him. Tell him what you want, and if he's not quick enough, push him to act faster. For example, if you want oral, tell him. If he doesn't perform the way you want, press his face into you, or better, roll him onto his back and ride his face. Just take care not to hurt him, and don't take it too far: some men don't like an overly dominant woman.

Play Damsel in Distress

As an alternative to the dominant woman, let him be the dominant man. Play the damsel in distress and let him come to your rescue. Or, be downright submissive. You can start by calling him something like "master" or "daddy" and letting him know you're at his service. Men love the way this type of role play enhances their ego and makes them feel more manly and strong. It plays on their basic instinct to want to be your protector and your dominant.

Pleasuring Her

Unlike men, women are more stimulated mentally. This can seem daunting, but it's really easy. In fact, it opens the door for many more ways to pleasure a woman and get her turned on.

Things as simple as complimenting her in a way you don't normally do can start the fire. Here are some more ways you can get her going:

Talk to Her

Women can be turned on solely through talk if you play your cards right. There are many things you can say to a woman to turn her on. Y

ou can: compliment her, admire her, tell her what you want to do to her, demand her to do something to you (if she's into that), and more. Use a low and commanding voice when you're speaking, and sometimes say them quietly in her ear. Try any of these things, and we guarantee you will have her quivering in no time.

Massage her Breasts, Butt, or Thighs

Stimulation is important to women; it helps turn them on and get them ready for what's to come. Adequate stimulation is what helps a woman produce her own lubricant to make sex pleasurable for her: if she isn't wet enough, it will probably just hurt. While there are several areas on a woman's body that can be touched, rubbed, or gently squeezed to turn her on, the best ones are her breasts, her butt, and her thighs. These areas tend to send electricity throughout her entire body.

Use your Touch

When you're giving compliments and making out with her, try pressing your hand into her thigh, or holding the small of her back. You can also: stroke her cheek, hold the back of her neck and pull her in closer for the kiss, hold her shoulder, or press other parts of your body into her. The idea is to physically stimulate her while also giving her the feeling that you can't get close enough, and you want to fully embrace her.

Undress her

Don't let your lady undress herself. In fact, bonus points if you don't let her take anything off of her own body. Slowly undress her, taking each item off and laying it next to the bed for her. Trace her body while you're doing this, and gently caress and kiss each part of her body that is being exposed. Be gentle during this time, it will make her feel like a queen.

Take your Time

Foreplay is the most important for women. As previously mentioned, if a woman isn't adequately turned on before sex, she will not be wet enough to accommodate for you. It will likely just be an unpleasant experience for the both of you, and who wants that? For her sake and yours, take your time! It will blow her mind that you care enough to make sure she is enjoying herself just as much as you are.

Nibble Her
Gentle nibbles in the right areas can send sparks through a lady's body.

Try nibbling her sensitive areas such as her breasts, her ears, her thighs, her bum, or her neck. Take care to be gentle though: outright biting can be painful and ruin the mood. Unless she's into that, of course.

Oral Foreplay
Oral sex is one of the best ways to turn your partner on. While it may seem very straight forward, there are many tips and tricks to help increase the pleasure your partner gains from your oral treat. Below, we have provided all of the best tips and tricks for orally stimulating your partner's genitals.

Blow Jobs
When you're pleasuring your man, offering a blow job is one of the best ways to get him rock hard and ready for sex. While it might seem straight forward: open your mouth and suck, there are many things you can do to step up your game and maximize the experience for both of you.

Get dramatic about it
before you go down on him, get him ready. Kiss your way down his body, run your hands down his chest.

Be Controlling
don't ask if he wants a blow job, just give him one. Pull his hands away, grab his dick and go to town.

Take Your Time
don't rush it: your rhythm can be slow, and the blow job should last a while. Don't go so long that he cums before sex, but definitely bring him to the edge before stopping.

Explore

you don't have to restrict your mouth to his shaft. Explore his balls, his frenulum and even take some time to nibble on his inner thighs.

Eye Contact

there is something extremely sexy about looking someone in the eye while they satisfy you with oral sex. Make sure you look up every now and again to meet his eye contact. You'll also love seeing how much he is enjoying himself.

Get Rough

not with his penis, that will hurt. But try digging your nails into his bum, or dragging them along the backs of his legs.

Flick Your Tongue

use the tip of your tongue and flick it around his penis, or lick it like you're eating ice cream.

Using different levels of suction and more or less tongue can create all kinds of sexy sensations that arouse him and get him ready for you.

Take It Slow

you don't have to consume his entire shaft in one go, right off the bat. In fact, if deep throating isn't you're thing, you don't have to do it at all. While some guys love the sight (and sound) of their lady gagging on him, the experience should be enjoyable for you, too. Take it inch by inch, and don't go any deeper if it becomes uncomfortable.

Encourage Him to Take Control

you can take his hands and guide them to your hair and encourage him to take hold and guide you onto his penis. From there, let him have control over the depth and speed at which you blow him. Just, make sure he's aware of your boundaries beforehand. You can also place your hands on his thighs so you can press your head backwards if you need him to go more shallow for you.

Hide

to boost the sexiness of your blow job, try hiding from him while you do it! You can either go under the blanket, or get him under the table for a naughtier experience. He will love that he has no idea what to expect!

The Art of Kissing

Kissing is seen as something that should occur prior to sex, and Vatsyayana was a firm believer that actions such as kissing, embracing, and scratching are not meant to be used during sexual intercourse. Instead, these are all different forms of foreplay, and as such, should be engaged in with the intention of arousing our partner and preparing them for a sexual union. Where you can kiss on a person's body is virtually limitless, but in the Kama Sutra, there are strict rules about where is acceptable and where is not. The places listed as acceptable to kiss are:

- The forehead

- The eyes

- The cheeks

- The lips

- Inside the mouth

- The throat

- The chest

- The breasts

Beyond this, the rest of the body is listed as off-limits to kissing, although the author does mention that some regions around the world do also allow for kissing on:

- The thighs

- The arms

- The belly button

It is very important that each person pays close attention to where their partner prefers to be kissed so that they may please them and not cause any distress. Kissing involves the use of your mouth, which is one of the most sensitive parts of the body. You could use your lips or tongue to lick, suck, kiss, and nibble or nozzle areas on your partner's body. Kissing is even art of its own you and your partner can use every day. And Kama Sutra recognizes the benefits of kissing and its different forms. The intensity of the way you kiss your partner has a role it plays on expressing your feelings to your partner. The intensity of a kiss uses a combination of three senses - smell, taste, and touch — each of these parts of the body produces a strong emotional response from your partner. Kissing ranges from fleeting contact to deep penetration with your tongue and so on. Let's dive into it a little bit more.

Types of kissing

There are different types of kissing teachings from the Kama Sutra we would be featuring. You can learn from them and apply then to express a lifting in your relationship. Here are the different types of kissing.

The Bent Kiss

Why not kiss your lover naturally today with this bent kiss. With your head angled slightly on one side which will allow you to get a maximum lip contact. You can even have a deep tongue penetration with this type of kiss, which is very sensual.

To perform this type of kiss, gently approach your partner and draw it very slowly as you head tilt to one side. You can pick any side you like - left or right. As you go for the kiss, take it slowly, let the lips touch first then after the full contact you then open your lips and play around with it before going for the deep penetration. You can also place your hand at the back of your partners head as you rub it gently for a more sensual feeling.

The Turned Kiss

If you want to tease your lover and make them feel gentleness and tenderness go for this type of kiss. This type of kiss is also perfect when you want to start foreplay with your partner. Also when you're making love slowly in a face-to-face standing or sitting position.

To perform this type of kiss, one of you, preferable the man turns up the face of his love by holding the chin and head. In that position, he then goes in slowly as your lips touch hers.

The Straight Kiss

When you kiss your love with your heads, you wouldn't be able to have so much of the tongue penetration. This kiss isn't to express an intense passion but a gentle way of showing affection and expression of desire. This type of kiss is recommended for new lovers.

To perform this type of kiss, let your lover sits on your laps and uses your hand to caress, fondle, her body, especially her back while kissing. Then as you go for the kiss, let your heads be angled only slightly, that it would seem almost straight. Then let your lips come in direct contact with each other and enjoy yourself.

Pressed Kiss

This type of kiss is more of an erotic prelude to kissing. It's sensual as you'd feel the contact of your lovers lips. There are two ways you can have this kiss with your lover.

The first method is when you are kissing your lover, and you press your lover's lower lips with force. This kiss expresses the degrees of passion you feel for your lover at that moment. And if you do it right, it can prelude to even more foreplay and clothes go off, and you know the rest.

For the second method, you use your lips to touch your loves lower lips first, then you go for a greatly pressed kiss. This other type of kiss is even more emotional than the first one, so you can choose any one of the two types of pressed kisses to show how much passion is in your heart.

Kissing the Upper Lips

This kissing from the teaching in Kama Sutra, Vatsyayana talks about a woman returning a man's kiss, making it clear that a woman can also initiate the kiss. This can also apply to other forms of lovemaking. So, women shouldn't feel afraid to make the first move.

To perform this kiss, as you kiss your lover's upper lips, she returns the kiss by kissing his lower lip. You can increase the sensuality of the kiss by kissing your partner's upper and lower lips in turn. And like most kisses, you and your lover can have it sitting, standing or lying down.

The Clasping Kiss

This type of kiss is the one where either the woman or man takes both the lips of the other between her or his lips. However, for the woman, you can only enjoy taking this kiss when your lover doesn't have a mustache. That way, you don't have to get all those hair in your mouth.

When you are enjoying this type of kiss with your lover and your lover uses his/her tongue to touch the tongue, teeth, or palate of your lover, it's called the fighting of the tongue. Generally, in clasping kiss, scrupulous oral hygiene is important.

A Young Girl's Kiss
The young girl's kiss is a type of kiss the Kama text recommend for lovers who are about to have sex for the first time. There are different types of young girl's kiss, and it's recommended that the kiss is done moderately and not to be continued for a long time.

The nominal kiss
to have this kiss like a girl, use your mouth to touch your love's own. But don't do the touching yourself, approach your lover closely, and he would do the touching himself.

The throbbing kiss
to have this kiss as a girl set your bashfulness aside touches the lips of her lover that is pressed into her mouth and with an object moves her lower lips but not the upper one.

The touching kiss
to have this kiss as the girl kiss your lover by using your tongue to touch his lips. As you close your eyes, place your hands on your lover's hands and enjoy the kiss.

Pressing of the Nails and Scratching
There are eight different types of scratches that are described within the Kama Sutra, each based on a certain way of pressing the nails into the skin.

Sounding
Pressing in the nails so that no mark is made

Half Moon
Leaving a curved mark along the neck and breasts

Circle
Two half-moons created beside each other

Line
A scratch that is made in the shape of a line

Tiger's Nail
A curved scratch made on the breast

Peacock's Foot
A curved mark made by pressing all 5 nails into the breast

The Jump of a Hare
A scratch-made with all 5 nails near the nipple

Leaf of a Blue Lotus
A mark made in the shape of a lotus near the breast

These marks are all designed to be placed in hidden locations across the body, particularly on the breast, so that they are only seen by the two lovers and by no one else. They are there to remind the person of their lover and to excite them whenever they gaze upon each mark.

Biting
Similar to the pressing of nails and scratching, there are eight different kinds of bites that are made by a lover onto the body of their partner. These are also done in private places on the body and are used as a way to remind the partner that they are loved and desired. The eight types of bites are:

Hidden Bite
A bite where no teeth marks are left, only redness in the area

Swollen Bite
When the bite causes the skin to be pressed on both sides

Point
Only two teeth are utilized in order to nip at a small section of skin

Line of Points
Using all of the teeth to bite at small sections of skin

Coral and the Jewel
When you bite someone using both your teeth and lips

Line of Jewels
Any bite that is made using all of the teeth

Broken Cloud
If you have space between your teeth, this type of bit will leave a round mark that is not fully enclosed

Biting of a Boar
Many rows of bites all close to one another

Striking
When it comes to striking a lover, this should only be employed during sex and with the consent of both individuals involved. Not everyone enjoys being slapped or struck, so never engage in this unless you have discussed it beforehand. If, however, both of you are interested in adding in striking during sexual intercourse, the Kama Sutra lays out the rules for doing so.

First, the places that you are allowed to strike your partner are:

- The head

- The shoulders

- The back

- The sides

- In between their breasts

- The Jaghana

You may then strike them in four different ways:

- With the back of your hand

- With the fingers sprawled out

- With an open hand

- With a fist

It is during being struck that a lover will make various sounds, as she may be in pain and so she will cry out. Any blows that one lover delivers, should always be reciprocated by the other. This is never a one-sided activity, and each action should be mirrored in order to highlight the pleasures that are being felt. It is also important that you strike in different ways along different spots on the body. For example, if striking with a fist, this should only be done along the back as it is sturdier and should never be done to the head. Striking should never be done in excess and is not done out of anger but instead out of pure pleasure.

CHAPTER 5

EMOTIONAL VS PHSYCAL INTIMACY

Intimacy is oftentimes confused with something that is sexual in nature, when in fact intimacy can be displayed in both asexual and non-sexual manner. Friends can be intimate with one another, you can have an intimate relationship with an individual who is not a lover, a certain setting, mood, or location can be intimate, and as most of us are aware, we can have an intimate relationship with our spouse or lover.

Simply put, intimacy is the closeness that you feel with another person and exists within all types of loving relationships. In a non-human sense, intimacy can also be felt in cozy, private settings such as an intimate concert, or intimate dining experience. For the purpose of this chapter, however, we will be focusing on the intimacy felt between two people, particularly lovers, and how to ignite and increase it.

Within intimacy there are four distinct types:

- Physical

- Emotional

- Intellectual

- Experiential

Each one needs to be nurtured within a relationship in order to make it successful, for it is through intimacy that we develop vulnerability, closeness, a feeling of being connected, and a healthier experience. But how exactly do we go about increasing our intimacy? Below we will look at the different ways the Kama Sutra suggests increasing intimacy via touch both by embracing in different ways, as well as through the art of kissing.

Kama Sutra Embraces

Within the Kama Sutra, there are different types of embraces listed that explain in detail how we can hold someone to us. Four of the embraces listed are non-sexual, while the other four are sexual in nature. These unique styles of embracing increase both intimacy and passion and can physically connect two people so that they feel closer to one another both literally and metaphorically speaking. Beyond the eight standard embraces, the Kama Sutra also lists an additional four that forgo the use of the arms and instead focuses on embracing using other parts of the body. In this way, the book goes into great detail on all of the ways in which we can use our bodies to show our love to one another.

Since the Kama Sutra does have a focus on sexual acts, the type of intimacy created through these embraces is one that is more sexual in nature. But, not all of the embraces should be done during a session of passionate lovemaking, and instead, some of the options listed are to be engaged in between individuals who are not yet actively intimate and instead are getting to know each other beforehand. By embracing someone you are letting your guard down and physically letting them enter into your space. You are welcoming them to get to know your body, as well as who you are in the process. Embracing is a very intimate act, and below we will look at the different types and who they should be done by. The first four embraces listed are external embraces, otherwise known as preparatory embraces.

They are to be used between a couple who has come to love one another and are done prior to intercourse although not necessarily as foreplay. Instead, they heighten the intimacy felt between the couple, as well as arouse the man and create an erection.

Sprishtaka – The Touching or Contact Embrace

The first type of embrace listed in the Kama Sutra is the Touching Embrace and it is recommended to be done by individuals who are not yet in a relationship and instead are courting or flirting with one another. This is the least sexual of the embraces and is the common form of hugging that we know today. The Kama Sutra describes it as an action in which a man stands in front of a woman, or to the side of her, and then touches her body with his. He may wrap his arms around her, one arm around her, or simply touch her with as much body contact as possible.

Viddhaka – The Piercing or Bruising Embrace

The second embrace that is designed for couples who are not yet in a sexual relationship but moving towards it, is the Piercing Embrace. This should be done only in a private setting as it is more intimate in nature than the Touching Embrace. This embrace happens when a woman bends over as if she is about to pick something up, and in the process, she pierces a man with her breasts. The man can either be sitting or standing, so long as her breasts hit against him. In response to her action, the man should then grab ahold of her breasts and embrace them.

Uddhrishtaka – The Rubbing or Baring Embrace

This embrace is the first listed that should only be done between individuals who are already open about their intentions with one another and who speak freely about their feelings. This type of embrace occurs either in a public setting or in private, but always when two lovers are walking with each other slowly in the dark. It is here that they should rub their bodies together intimately, creating the Rubbing Embrace.

Piditaka – The Pressing or Squeezing Embrace

Closing out the first four External or Preparatory embraces is the Pressing Embrace. Like with the Rubbing Embrace, this occurs when two lovers are walking together in public or private under the fall of darkness. When they come upon a wall or a pillar, one person should forcibly press the other against it and then the man can press his erection against the woman's body. This is an ideal transition embrace from the External section into the Preliminary Love Play embraces, as it involves the man being erect and can thus lead to sexual intercourse. Preliminary love play is commonly referred to as foreplay, and Vatsyayana details four distinct embraces that should be used during this period. The first two of the embraces are meant to occur when both lovers are standing up. The final two are meant to be used during the act of lovemaking, which contradicts the fact that they are listed under preliminary embraces as they technically would not occur beforehand. However, as you read the descriptions, you should see that no mention of sex is actually listed, so it would seem that all four can actually be used to create intimacy prior to, as well as during, sex.

Jataveshtitaka – The Twining of a Creeper

The name of this embrace makes it sound creepy, but a creeper is like a vine that winds its way around a tree. So is this embrace, as the woman winds her way around the man and holds onto him closely. For the Twining of a Creeper, a woman should wrap her body around his man in whatever way she sees fit, embracing him while staring at him in a loving manner. She should take his head and bend it down towards her as if she is asking for a kiss, then make the sound of 'sut sut'. While all of this is happening, the couple is engaged in the Twining of a Creeper.

Vrikshadhirudhaka – Climbing a Tree
The second embrace that is listed as one that should occur during preliminary love play is Climbing a Tree. Also done while standing, this embrace features the woman standing with one of her feet placed on top of the foot of her lover, and her second foot pressed onto his thigh. She should then take one arm and wrap it around his back, which her other armrests on his shoulders. The sounds she makes will be that of singing as well as a cooing noise. It is called Climbing a Tree because it as if she wishes to climb up the man in order to kiss him and become intimate.

Tila Tandulaka – The Mixture of Sesamum Seed with Rice
The following two embraces are both listed as ones that should be done at the time of sexual intercourse. As you will notice, both can either be done right before you begin or even utilized during the act to draw you and your lover closer together. In this first embrace, both partners should be laying down in bed in order to begin. Here, the man and woman will entangle themselves within each other by embracing so tightly that each arm encircles the others, while each thigh is wrapped against their partner's. The Kama Sutra goes on to specify that if a man is laying down on his right-hand side, then he should take his left leg and put it in between the woman's thighs. Then, with his left arm, he will wrap it around the woman's right side.

Kshiraniraka – Milk and Water Embrace
The final embrace that is featured under Preliminary Love Play is the Milk and Water Embrace. Mentally, the couple should be in a space where they are both deeply and truly in love and

where nothing else matters to either of them. If this is their mindset, then they should embrace as tightly as possible, almost as if their bodies are attempting to merge into one another. This can be done in any position, either with the woman sitting on the man's lap, sitting in front of each other, or laying down in bed. There are four final embraces that do not involve the use of the arms, and instead are focused on various body parts embracing one another. These embraces can be used during foreplay or during the course of sex as they mostly are comprised of ways of pressing against your lover.

The Embrace of the Thighs

For the Embrace of the Thighs, one partner will take the other's thighs between their own and squeeze them tightly. They can either focus on one of their lover's thighs, or they can place both between their legs.

Jaghana – The Embrace of the Sexual Area

Jaghana refers to the sexual area of the body that exists below the belly button but above the thighs. Both the genital area as well as the anal area are included in this section. For the Embrace of the Sexual Area, the woman will lay on her back with the man laying flat on top of her. Here he will imitate the act of sex by pressing his genitals down against her. He can then engage in any number of sexually motivated actions, such as scratching, biting, slapping, kissing, or playing with the woman's long and flowing hair.

Embrace of the Breasts

The Embrace of the Breasts occurs when a man takes his chest and presses it firmly between the woman's breasts. This can occur while standing or laying down, but simply means that both individuals are tightly embraced chest to chest. There does not need to be any other body parts involved, including the arms, in order to engage in the Embrace of the Breasts.

Embrace of the Forehead

The final embrace that is described within the Kama Sutra is the Embrace of the Forehead. This involves both partners placing their foreheads against one another, while also touching together their mouth and eyes. Intimate and sensual, this is a very passionate embrace that leads perfectly into our next section regarding the different ways in which we kiss.

Emotional Vs. Physical Intimacy

In this section, I am going to define emotional and physical intimacy before comparing the two in a variety of ways.

Emotional intimacy is the ability to express oneself in a mature and open manner, which leads to a deep emotional connection between two people. Saying things like "I love you" or "you are very important to me" are examples of this. It is also the ability to respond in a mature and open way when someone expresses themselves to you by saying things like "I'm sorry" or "I love you too." This type of intimacy is found in romantic relationships and in some friendships or familial relationships.

Physical intimacy is the type of intimacy that most people think of when they hear the term, and it is the kind that we have been addressing the most so far in this book. This is the type of intimacy that includes physical touch, including sex and all activities related to sex. However, it also involves other non-sexual types of physical contact such as hugging and kissing.

How to Increase Intimacy

In a romantic or sexual relationship, intimacy is a given. You would not enter a romantic relationship without some degree of emotional intimacy, and a sexual relationship by definition involves physical intimacy. For a romantic relationship to be successful, both forms of intimacy must be present between the partners. Without intimacy, there is nothing that sets a romantic relationship apart from an everyday friendship. Intimacy is something that must be worked at and maintained consistently, especially emotional intimacy. In a romantic relationship, however, physical intimacy must be maintained as well as this is one way of showing the other person that you feel strongly for them. If intimacy is lacking or if it fades over time, there are some things that you can do to revive or rekindle it.

The first way to restore intimacy in a relationship or to develop it in the first place is through communication. Communication is key in a relationship of any sort, but especially in a romantic relationship. Communicating is the only sure way to know where the other person stands in terms of their thoughts and feelings. Being able to be vulnerable and open with your emotions is a requirement for intimacy. It is necessary to share oneself with the other person in a relationship. This mutual sharing of yourselves is what will lead to intimacy in the first place or an increase in intimacy.

It is important to communicate about your needs for intimacy on a recurring basis since people will grow and change over the course of a relationship. Especially in a long-term relationship, being aware of when a person's intimacy needs change is important to maintaining a good level of intimacy.

When working on intimacy, it is helpful to start slow by talking about things that are easier for you to open up about-like your future goals or your ideal job. This is still a way to open up without pushing yourself too far right away. It can be scary to be that vulnerable with someone. It is also helpful to note that for many people, there are things that they consciously avoid thinking about, as they may be painful to address. It will be very difficult for them to voice these things to themselves, so allow them to start slowly and don't be offended if you feel like there are topics that they are uncomfortable talking about.

Many people have a fear of intimacy, and this is also worth noting. Because intimacy needs trust in order to develop, it can be hard for some people who have had past experiences that make it hard for them to trust people. By being aware of this, it may help you to understand why your partner has trouble opening up. It may also help you if you have a fear of intimacy as you can explain this to your partner in order to ask for the patience you will need as you begin to open up and be vulnerable with them.

When it comes to improving intimacy, it is a slow build and not a race to the finish line. Be patient with yourself and your partner, and try to see intimacy as a growing experience between you that will continue throughout the entire duration of your relationship.

Best Positions for Intimacy

Sex also happens to come with many other benefits, but these positions we will explore now are chosen because they are the best for creating intimacy and connection for you and your partner.

The Lotus

Arguably the most intimate position of them all is The Lotus. The Lotus position is most intimate because of the closeness of your entire bodies, infinitely pressed against each other at all points from head to toe while being face to face.

The man sits on the bed cross-legged, his torso upright. His penis is erect and ready to get it on. The woman climbs on top of him and sits in his lap, wrapping her arms and legs around him. He holds her by wrapping his arms around her as well.

With some shifting, they slide his penis inside of her. In this position, both people will be grinding more than they will be thrusting or humping. This is also what makes it so intimate. Grinding face to face while she is sitting on his lap with him inside of her, that is about as intimate as it gets.

In this position, you will not be doing any crazy thrusting, so it is ideal for a steamy make-out session, as your mouths will be so close that you can feel each other's breath the entire time. You can look into each other's eyes and whisper sweet nothings to them as you share this intimate experience.

Slow Grind

Another position that makes for a high level of intimacy and closeness is the Slow Grind position. In this position, the man sits down with his legs extended and leans back on his hands. The woman climbs on top of him, facing him and puts his penis inside of her. she extends her legs past him and leans back on her hands as well. In this position, they cannot move too much without risking his penis sliding out of her, so they are restricted to a slow grind. They both slowly grind their hips into each other and move gently. With both of their arms occupied to hold them up, they can only move their hips, and this makes for an intimate mood with no distractions of arms and legs moving about. They are seated facing each other as well, so they will look at each other in the eyes as they slowly grind and pleasure each other. You can see why this position is such an intimate one for a couple to try together.

CHAPTER 6:

THE TOP POSITIONS

Beginners

Missionary Position

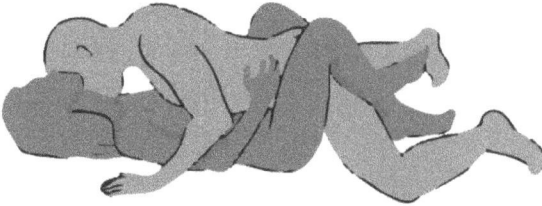

A lso known as the 'classic', the missionary position is the most commonly used technique for couples today. It hardly requires an illustration and typically used because it is very comfortable for the female (and the male gets to do all the work!). Unfortunately, the pace and strength of the sex is left mainly for the male so with an unskilled lover, it's unlikely that a girl will reach orgasm.

This is why guys who prefer the missionary position but want to provide their partners with as much pleasure as possible are advised to do more with their hands and mouth. Missionary typically requires that the whole male body is plastered to the female body, crushing the breasts and keeping the pelvis in close contact with each other. If this is the case, make sure to ground the pelvis to the clitoris as much as possible, imitating a grinding-circular motion to really hit the clitoris and the U-Spot. Utilizing the mouth to bite, suckle, and lick the erogenous zones like the neck, the nape, the lips, and the nipples will also add to the female's pleasure.

Concealed Door
In this position, the female lays completely on her front as the male mounts her from the back. He covers her with his whole body as the penis penetrates from the back, the male legs and elbows used to prevent his body weight from completely crushing the female. In this position, the male moves back and forth and use his hands to caress the breast. He may also kiss and suck her nape or perform other methods of additional stimulation.

Doggy Style
The doggy style is a favorite for many guys because it offers incredibly deep penetration. Women also find this an excellent technique because it helps hit more pleasurable spots in the vagina. Depending on the angle of the penetration, doggy style can hit the P-Spot or the G-Spot, both of which are highly sensitive. Even if these two spots aren't stimulated however, guys have the option of stimulating the clitoris, the U-Spot, and the K-Spot using their hands. Women can also use their fingers to add to the pleasure by stroking the clitoris. Hence, it's a position of infinite possibilities and with just a few tweaks, can further heighten the pleasure.

There are essentially two ways to perform the doggy style. The first one is common whereby the women goes on all fours and spreads her legs wide for penetration. The second technique is when the female keeps her thighs close together. Either position allows the female to keep both hands stretched out or flat on her chest. Of the two, the closed thighs position is often more pleasurable for the male because it grips the penis tighter.

The Split

The split is another fairly common sex position that allows sufficient room for additional stimulation.

The male straddles one of the female's thighs while draping the other on his shoulders.

This allows for a deep penetration while leaving the hands free to play with the clitoris or the breasts. Most of the pace and thrusts is controlled by the male as the female lies back and enjoys the ride.

Girls can also try stroking themselves or the penis as it moves back and forth. With this position, guys can enjoy the motion of the breasts as it bobs up and down.

The Cowgirl

The cowgirl leaves most of the work for the girl as she chooses the depth and pacing that offers her the most pleasure. The downside is that its hell on the legs – but you'll definitely be trimming some fat in your thighs with this move.

The guy lies down on his back as the girl straddles him for a ride. The classic cowgirl typically means that the girl is facing forward, allowing the male to enjoy her breasts.

If your partner is an ass-man however, the reverse cowgirl would be better.

Depending on the position, the male can play with the clitoris or the K-Spot as the female bounces on top.

Against the Wall

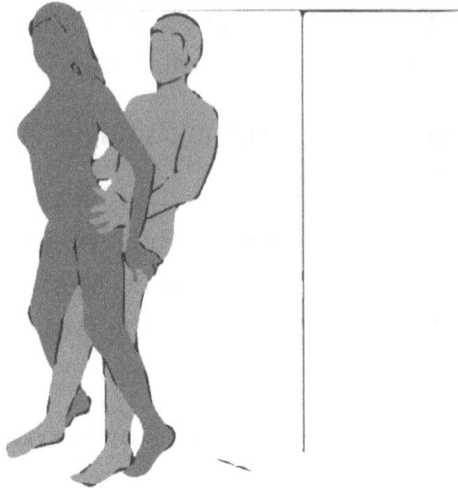

No image necessary since against the wall sex is pretty common for couples nowadays. Unfortunately, most couples don't utilize the full potential of this position for pleasure. There are essentially two ways to perform this technique. The female can either be facing the wall or leaning against it.

Leaning against the wall, the girl can lift one foot onto the male's hip and use the other one for leverage so that she can also help control the thrust and pace during sex. In this position, one of the guy's hands can be used to provide support for the raised leg while the other performs more pleasurable activities like stroking the K-Spot. In this position, the male can also play with the breast using his tongue or go for other erogenous zones like the neck, the ears, and the lips. Guys who have the muscle strength for it can wrap the girl's thighs around their waist, leaving them full control on the thrusts.

The female can also face the wall, using both hands as a way to balance themselves as well as help control the movement during sex. This is basically a doggy style position standing up, letting men use the boobs as handles as they control the sex. In this position however it's usually better to play with the clitoris since you get maximum access in this situation. Some women find it more pleasurable to have their front smashed against the wall, crushing the breasts with each thrusting motion.

Mare's Position

The final technique that is listed under Low Congress in the Kama Sutra is the Mare's Position. Like we saw with The Pressing Position and the Twining Position, this is in fact not a position at all and is instead a way for the woman to increase tightness during sex.

What is required here is for the woman to literally trap the man's lingam inside her yoni so that he cannot remove himself. This is going to require the woman to have developed her Kegel muscles so that they are able to be engaged at her will. The Kama Sutra does make a point of saying that this technique is only learned through practice and is performed only by certain women who have been trained in this act.

If you want to be able to engage in The Mare's Position during sex, then you are going to need to train yourself to be able to utilize your Kegel muscles when you like. You will also need to practice strengthening them, as simply squeezing gently will not be enough to trap the man's penis inside you.

In order to strengthen these particular muscles, you will need to learn exactly what you are feeling for, and this can be done the next time you go to urinate.

While peeing, stop yourself mid-stream by clenching your pelvic muscles, then release and continue urinating. Once you have the hang of this, you can then practice that same motion anywhere and anytime.

You should hold the muscles tightly for 3 to 5 seconds at a time, and then release them for 3 to 5 seconds. Repeat these multiple times a day, for at least 10 times per session. For those that want to take their practice a step further, you can actually invest in devices that are designed specifically for this purpose. Yoni eggs are small ball-shaped items that are placed inside the vagina that you can practice squeezing tightly.

The benefits of strengthening your Kegel muscles extend far beyond The Mare's Position, however, and this is actually something all women should practice doing.

Strong Kegel muscles can help prevent incontinence as you age, or that can develop from pregnancy and birth. This also strengthens the pelvic floor which can aid in childbirth, as well as preventing the pelvic floor from collapsing post-birth.

Kneeling Fox
The kneeling fox is a spin-off of the classic doggy-style. This position allows for him to penetrate her deeply, while going as fast or as slow as he wants.

She can also grind her hips back to meet his thrusts and further deepen the penetration. It works by having the gentleman sit on the bed on his knees.

Then, the lady squats on all fours, then sits back on his lap. He can then hold her hips as leverage, while she grinds her hips backwards to meet his thrusts. T

his will help increase the level of penetration and help her gain control on where he is stimulating her.

Standing Spoon

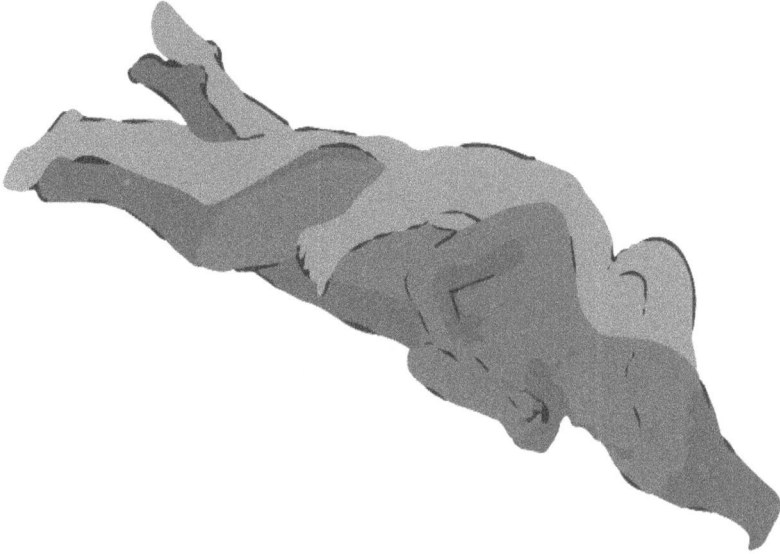

This sex position involves both parties standing up. It works best in a hall way, or at least next to a wall for balance. To start, you want to have the man behind the woman, holding her by the hips.

Then, she can stand in front of him, and lean forward slightly. He can proceed to enter her from behind, while one or both of you use the walls for balance and leverage.

Also, this position is excellent for allowing both parties to have control over the speed and depth of penetration.

The Scissors

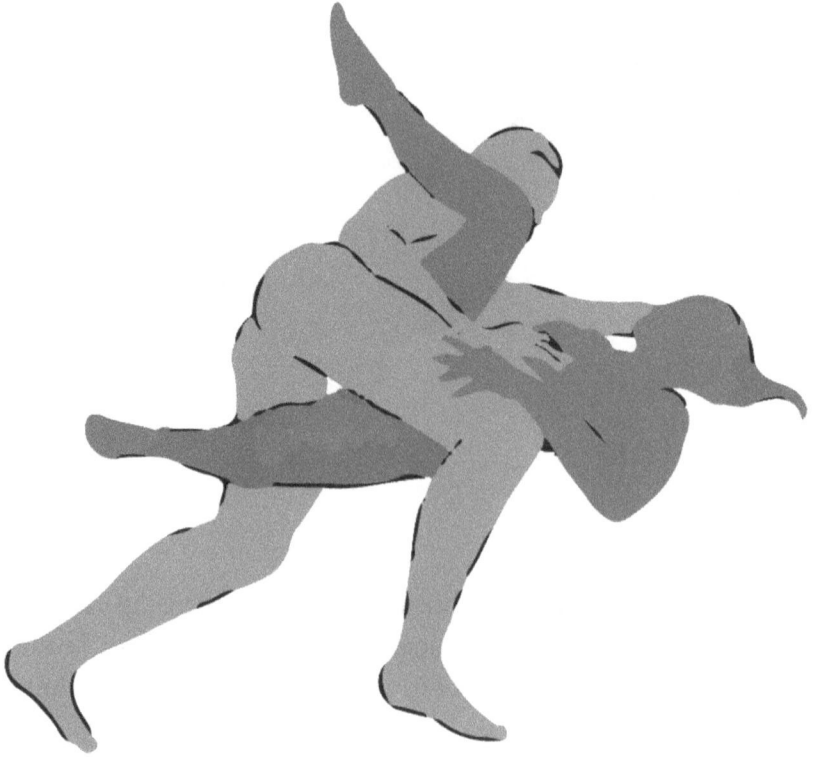

This is a reversal on the sexy spoons, and allows for both lovers to have some intimate face-to-face time. It is great for making out during sex, or having some deep eye gazing. To start, both the gentleman and lady should be lying on the bed facing each other. Then, she should put her leg over top of his hip, while he grabs her bum. Your bottom legs should be pressed together, and then you achieve penetration front-to-front. Using each other's hips as leverage, you can both control the speed and rhythm by which you're moving.

Intermediate

Climbing the Tree

Requiring balance from both the male and the female, Climbing the Tree is basically standing sex without the benefit of a wall. According to the Kama Sutra, this position provides a different kind of orgasm due to the sexual pleasure along the spine. In this situation, the male is the Tree that the female climbs with the penis acting as a branch that prevents her from falling. One of the girl's legs is hitched around the hips of the male while the other maintains balance. In this position, the male is free to play with the K-Spot, stimulate the breasts with his mouth or engage in all manners of kissing and licking.

Almost 69

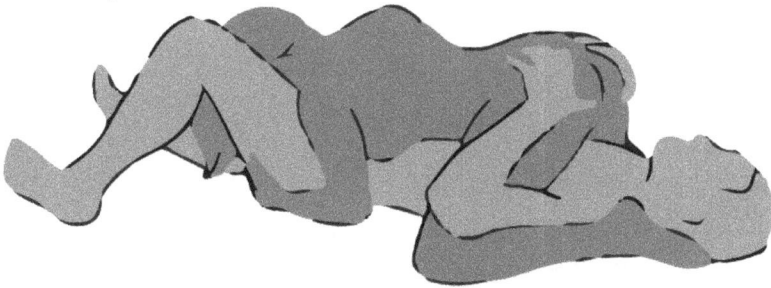

This position starts off like the Reverse Cowgirl but instead of the female staying upright, she continues to lie down to her stomach so that her face faces the feet of the male. In this position, both the girl and the boy control the movement as the female hooks her arms around the male's calves for leverage. The guy can hold onto the girl's hips to enforce more control and guide the rhythm and depth. For guys who love female ass, this is an ideal position – not to mention the fact that it lets them see the in and out movement of the penis. The only spot the guy can hit during the Almost 69 is the K-Spot although the girl can make an effort to brush her clitoris against the male with the movement.

The Lotus

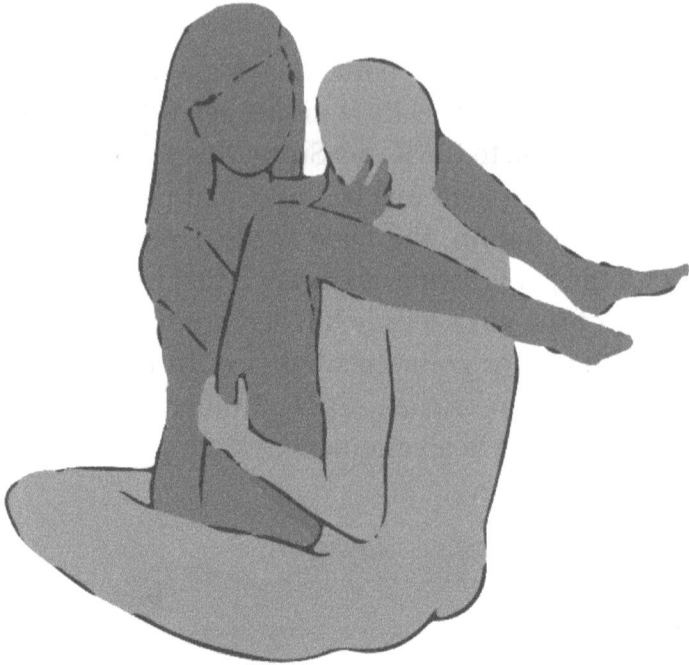

Most sexual positions require the female to be flexible but in the lotus, the male must be able to open his legs wide in a lotus position. If you've seen the position of the legs during yoga, this is exactly how it looks. The female then straddles the male, her breasts meeting his chest and getting as close as possible to effect penetration. The female wraps her thighs around the male as he controls the movement of the thrust. Women can also choose to brace their feet on the floor to help with the movement. In this position, guys can easily suck on the breasts, play with the K-Spot or perhaps do lots of smooching as they try to capture a steady rhythm to capture an orgasm. It can be tough for the guy but the open leg approach offers a different kind of pleasure for the lady. In this position, the head of the penis also gets lots of attention.

The Turning Position

When couples are making love, alternating the position can help to make lovemaking more intense and sensual as well as increase closeness. The turning position is a perfect type of love, making that is perfect for this kind of feeling. To have the turning position lovemaking with your lover, have a couple of foreplay to make the woman end up with her back on the bed. Then as the man fix yourself in-between her legs and go for the insertion. The lovemaking is more like the popular missionary lovemaking, but it comes with a twist. During lovemaking, the man can change position by lifting one of his legs and turn around without withdrawing from her. There are different ways the man can turn around in this position. There are about four different stages in this turning position.

The first stage is just like what I just explained above, the regular missionary position. The woman can caress and stroke the chest of her lover to give him more arousal, which can be a tricky maneuver. For the second stage, the man would lift his left leg and then his right leg to his lover's right leg and should not withdraw his penis from her vaginal.

The third stage involves the man moving both of his legs around, and this time, he does it without withdrawing his penis. He should make sure his body is at the right angle with his lover. Her legs also should be slightly apart as it would make it easier for him to keep his penis inside her vagina. And for the woman, she should lie back and enjoy the unusual angle of penetration. And the last fourth position is when he makes a complete 180-degree rotation in the sense that his body is between her legs one leg on either side of her shoulders. Navigating through these four stages of sex position is a bit difficult. But with practice, you would become a master in it in no time.

The Woman on Top Position

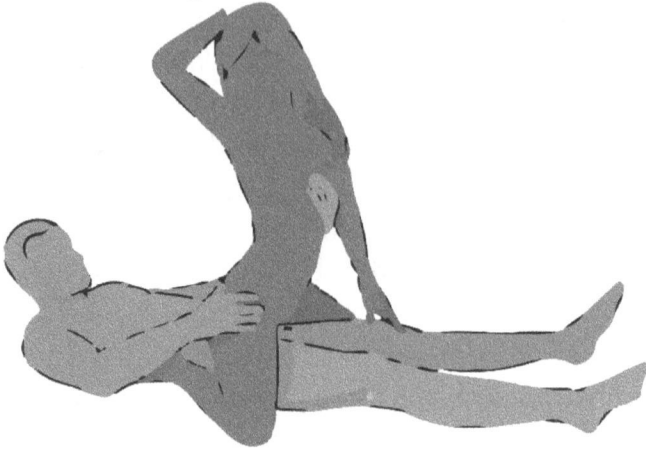

The woman on top is just like the turning position mentioned above, but this time around, the woman is on top of the man in this position. Again, it comes in three different stages which the woman can use to vary the position while making love to make lovemaking more fun. To have this form of lovemaking with your partner, the man should lie back down.

The woman would then cross her legs one on either side of the man. As she sits on her lover, they should both lock their fingers together. Then as she balances herself on her partner's lap, the congress should happen. While making love in this position, then you both should switch positions. The first stage is when the woman is in the normal facing her lover while they make love.

The second stage is when she tilts both of her legs to her lovers left side or right side depending on whichever side she prefers. She could keep her legs together for more sensual feeling as her vaginal would be tight. Or she could spread her legs to make the vaginal a little bit more open. She can then steady herself by putting a hand on his knee and the other hand on his chest for support.

The third and last stage is when the woman makes a full complete rotation where she now backs the man. She can place her hand on her lover's leg as she rides him. She could make movements like she's tweaking on his penis to make the sex faster and more sensual.

The Yawning Position
The yawning position is somewhat popular, but not everyone gets it right. This lovemaking position starts with a man in a more-or-less kneeling position. However, his knees should be widely spread. Not too wide, though! It should just be the right width for the woman to fit. Then the woman lying with her back on the bed raises her thigh and parts them on either side of the man. Her legs might get tired with time, so she can press her legs against his side to make it easier to keep them up. This position is pleasurable for both the man and the woman, but for the woman, it's all about getting the right thigh angle. Now, since the woman is lying down back on the bed, and the man on top (kneeling), pressing her thighs together, his side is an easy way to vary her thigh angle. Adjusting her thigh angle is also a way of varying the depth of penetration. Also, the barrier of the woman's thigh doesn't allow very deep penetration, but her clitoris gets much stimulation.

The man, on the other hand, should thrust himself forward gently against the woman's lower thigh for the penetration. He should also interlace his hands with the woman's hand to keep him up while penetrating. In general, this position is really erotic. Not to mention, her genitals are exposed, which turns the man on more. The helplessness she feels being on the bed in that locked position can also be a powerful turn on for both of them.

What you should note about this position is that her leg would feel a bit heavy with time since blood wouldn't flow much to her legs. So, don't use this position for a prolonged period. Also, since the man is somewhat resting on her hands, her hand would also feel tired at some point. Plus if you're a fan of fast sex, this position wouldn't really work for you. This position is for people who prefer a more gentle to a moderate speed of sex.

Stool Sex

Stool Sex works pretty much the same way as chair sex except the female's feet are planted firmly on the ground, her upper body bent downwards and holding onto a stool as the male enters her from behind. The lower height of the stool means the hips are tilted upwards, giving the guy one amazing angle to play with. Thrusting too much is not a good idea in this position since a stool isn't exactly a stable place for the girl to hold on to. On the plus side, this offers the guy a chance to hit that elusive G-Spot, especially if you happen to be long and thick. Couples who are into anal sex may also find this a favorite.

The Pressed Position

The Pressed Position was already mentioned above, when we discussed different ways you can utilize the Rising Position. Like previously described, this position involved the woman lying flat on her back, and then lifting her legs into the air. From here, she should place her legs on her man's shoulders in whatever position she finds most comfortable. Many women will perform this by simply placing their ankles on their partner's shoulders, while others will use their calves or the backs of their knees. Traditionally, this position has the woman resting her feet against the man's chest, a variation that narrows the vagina and makes more a more shallow but tight fit. Regardless of what you choose, as long as your legs or feet touch his shoulders you have successfully gotten into The Pressed Position.

This is such a popular position and many couples find it to be their favorite as it is extremely versatile. If you enjoy intimate sex, this position has you both gazing into other's eyes as he slowly works his way inside you. For those that prefer a much rougher and tumble version of sex, this pose will allow him to grip on to you and really go to work. No matter what your preference, this position can be adapted to suit almost any need and is sure to please both of you immensely.

The Posture of Splitting of a Bamboo

This is one of the first positions we are going to discuss that involves the woman actively participating in order to make it successful. With the Posture of Splitting a Bamboo, the woman will lay on her back with her partner kneeling in front of her. She will place one of her legs on his shoulders, and then stretch the other leg out to the side. The man should insert himself into the woman and begin having sex at this point. Now, here is where the woman will need to begin being more active. The leg that is on his shoulder, and the leg that is stretched out, will switch positions so that the stretched leg is now on his shoulder and the previously placed leg is now stretched out. Getting in rhythm with her man, the woman will continue to alternate her legs back and forth, keeping one on his shoulder and one outstretched at all times. The continuous movement of the legs will alter the angle of the vagina and change the sensation for the man, as well as change which part of the vagina is being hit with every thrust. We advise starting out slowly with this move until you feel more comfortable and confident. Not only is it difficult to constantly move your legs into different positions, but it can also be hard to time your movements with your man's thrust. The slower you start this, the easier of a time you will have, and you can build up speed as you go. Timing is everything with The Posture of Splitting of a Bamboo, and the more in sync you and your partner are, the better this will feel.

The Fixing of a Nail

Like with The Position of Splitting of a Bamboo, The Fixing of a Nail is another position that involves the woman moving her legs during sex. What makes this one different, however, is the fact that it requires a significant amount of flexibility on the woman's part, and it is unlikely that this position is going to be for everyone. Many thinks of the Kama Sutra as being a book of outrageous sex positions, and this is one of the mentioned poses that will seem crazy to a lot of people. For this position, the woman will again begin by lying on her back, and her man should kneel in front of her. From here, the man will take on of her legs, lift it up, and then begin to move it into a split like position, where the foot is stretching back towards the woman's head. She should then rest her foot against the man's forehead, while keeping the other leg remaining on the ground straight out as normal. If this doesn't sound difficult enough, the position continues on by having the woman continuously switch which leg is flat on the ground and which has the foot placed on the man's forehead.

For positions such as The Fixing of a Nail, which are more complicated and require a lot of flexibility, you can start by only trying the first half and skip out on switching the legs throughout sex. Having your foot on your man's forehead is already going to be a challenge, so if you manage to get that far then give yourself a round of applause. For those that are able to get into and maintain this position, then feel free to try the full pose by swapping the legs throughout. The switching does enhance the position as it alters the angle of the pelvis and gives a new sensation with every move.

Experts

Wheelbarrow
You've probably heard of the wheelbarrow which is actually a classic when it comes to difficult sex. It requires strength, mainly on the part of the female because she'll be supporting herself largely on her arms as the male controls the thrusting movement of the sex. In the wheelbarrow, the female goes down on all fours as the male's stands on the back. He then lifts the legs of the female and enters her from behind in a standing position.

There are several variants to the wheelbarrow. The male can either be kneeling or standing up. Depending on his position, the female can stretch out both hands to hold herself upwards or simply use pillows under her chest area to lift herself up. The typical wheelbarrow position consists of the legs opened wide and stretched straight upwards as the male holds onto the hips to maintain position. However, women have the option of keeping their knees tucked in so that the legs are bent. For others, one leg may be stretched out while the other is bent and tucked forward. These changes in leg position helps control the depth, pace, and control of the male so women are perfectly free to grab whatever position they want.

Love Triangle
This sensual position allows for deep penetration, as well as maximum stimulation of the lady's g-spot and clitoris. It is a move that requires both lovers to be somewhat flexible, but can be altered to work for basically any level of flexibility. To do this move, you want to start by having the lady laying on her back with her feet up. Her right leg should then drop to the side, so it stretches out at an angle. Then, the gentleman should come up between her legs and put his left foot over her right thigh to get good leverage for his penetration. The gentleman has

almost full control of this position, but the lady can gently rock back and forth to meet his thrusts. Also, due to how open the position is, either the lady or the gentleman can use a free hand to stimulate her clitoris for added pleasure.

The Supported Congress

The Supported Congress is the first of the positions we have come to that gets both partners up and off of the ground. Here is a classic standing pose that is fairly simple and is modified depending on your personal preference. To perform The Supported Congress, have both partners stand face one another. From here, you only need to find something to support you; the Kama Sutra suggests using each other's bodies, a wall, or a pillar. How you engage in sex after this point is up to you. Some options include standing with both feet on the ground and then angling the pelvis so that the man can insert himself into the woman. Another option is to have the woman raise one of her legs up so that entry can be even easier.

One important thing to know with most standing positions is that height differences can really make or break what you are able to do. In many cases, the man is going to be taller than the woman, which means their pelvic regions generally will not line up perfectly. To combat this issue, utilize things around the house to bring the woman up to a taller stance. You can try wearing high heels or standing on the lower part of your staircase if you have one. You can also stand on cushions, a small stepping stool, or anything else that is stable and gives you enough of a boost to have sex more enjoyable.

Sensory Support

This move is a deeply erotic one that provides explosive pleasures for her, and deep penetration for him. Plus, it is one where you get to gaze into each other's eyes while going at it. It is a standing position that requires the man to have enough strength to carry the womans weight. If he cannot completely handle her weight, he should stand with a bed or other piece of furniture high enough for her feet to rest on, so she can assist in balancing the two of them. First, the gentleman should be standing (with his back to the furniture if necessary). Then, the lady should stand in front of him and he should pick her up. She can either proceed to wrap her legs around his back, or rest her feet on the furniture behind him for balance. Then, he can bear her weight while bouncing her up and down. It is definitely a highly pleasurable move for both parties involved.

Pinwheel

This fun position allows for you to be face-to-face without being directly in each other's face. It works by having the gentleman sit down and lean back slightly with his hands back on the bed. Then, he bends his legs and lets his knees fall to either side while his feet stay close together. The lady then squats over his penis and controls the penetration, while wrapping her legs behind his back and leaning back on her hands. She has the most control over the speed and rhythm, but he can add to it with his own thrusts.

Head Over Heels

This move requires the lady to have a significant amount of strength in her entire body, but particularly her upper body. It is excellent for deep penetration, and g-spot stimulation. This position is a semi-standing one, that can be done virtually anywhere. It starts by having a lady go down on all fours, supporting her upper half with her forearms on the ground. Then, the gentleman stands behind her, grabs her feet, and lifts her vagina to meet his penis. From there, he can penetrate her and work at whatever pace they can comfortably handle in that position.

Dolphin

Dubbed as the dolphin, this sex positions starts off looking easy but can actually be tough overtime.

The male is basically kneeling on the bed, his thighs and upper body held straight upwards.

The female is lying on her back as her hips are tilted upwards to straddle the male thighs and effect penetration.

As a result, the female is basically arching her back while keeping her shoulders flat on the bedroom.

The male handles the depth and penetration by holding onto her buttocks for balance.

Wheelbarrow

The wheelbarrow functions much like the reverse of the dolphin and is equally complicated. It starts off with the female going on all fours at the edge of the bed.

The then positions from behind and grabs her legs to put them around his thighs.

The tough part comes when the male basically coaxes the girl to move backward so that the lower half of her body is now off the bed and completely supported by the guy.

Using her hands, the female plants them on the bed as the male straddles her from behind, her legs and hips dangling off the edge. In this position, the guy again gets most of the work and doesn't leave any room for additional stimulation.

iding the Horse

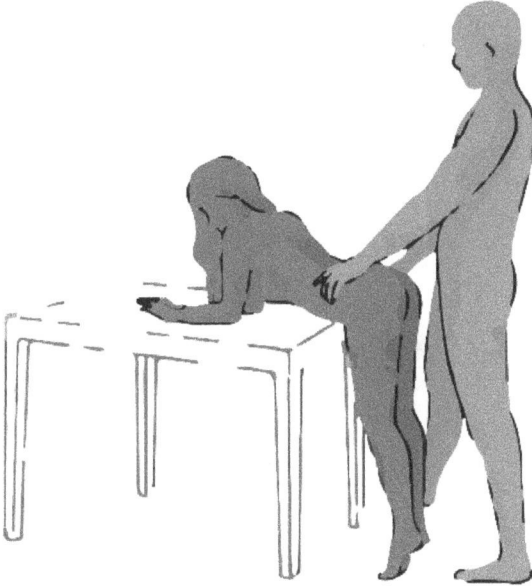

Definitely one of the most difficult sexual positions today, it's a little confusing why anyone would try doing this particular sex act – unless the couple is really into excitement. It works much like the Bridge which is illustrated below but is more precarious on the part of the girl. It starts off with the male supporting himself on his feet and hand in such a way that the penis is thrusting out upwards. The girl starts by straddling him from this position and then deftly lowers herself in such a way that one leg is between the thighs of the guy while the other is planted firmly on his upper body. The girl then leans backward and supports herself with one hand stretched out to the floor. In Riding the Horse, most of the job is done by the female since the male is mainly occupied with keeping himself upright. Undoubtedly, this position requires strength and stamina on both the girl and boy. On the plus side, it makes for an excellent core and arm exercise.

Bridge

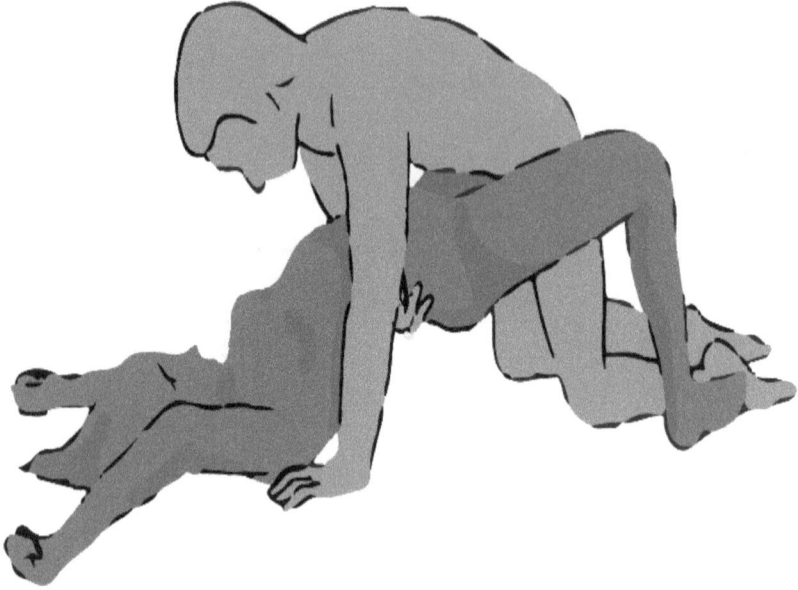

The bridge is terribly complicated and requires flexibility and strength from the guy. The male basically arranges himself into an arch; his body fully bending backwards until the only things supporting him is his hands and feet. The female then straddles him from this position and uses her leg for balance and leverage. The hands need to be used for additional balance so it's unlikely that the female would be able to pleasure herself using her hands. Still, it's an interesting position that should be tried out at least once.

CHAPTER 7:

THE TOP DOMINANTS POSITIONS

Men

The Pleasure Principle

Before explaining techniques on how a man can please a woman, the matter of how he learns must be addressed. While some men may have a selfish approach to sex, if a woman is learning about the Kama Sutra, it's a reasonable assumption that she is with a partner who cares aout her pleasure. That only leaves the question of whether or not her partner knows *how* to give her pleasure.

While learning techniques is always helpful, it is the woman's responsibility to communicate her desires and ways she enjoys being stimulated. For obvious reasons, it's to her benefit that she do so. Still, many women feel awkward, or fear their partner will think them "slutty" or "cheap". This is why it's so important to use the full scope of the Kama Sutra to create a deep connection. Any feelings of awkwardness or fear judgment must be addressed.

It's not fair for a partner to be limited in how much pleasure they can get from lovemaking because they're afraid to give a voice to their desires and fantasies. It's equally unfair to leave one's lover fumbling in the dark (sometimes literally!) to find what works and doesn't work for their partner.

Great sex requires the person feel sexy. And while being pleasured and desired can make a person feel sexy, they also need to feel they are good and pleasing their partner.

Some men don't take criticism well. But virtually all men want to be skilled lovers. So in order to educate them, it might come down to how the lesson is presented more than the lesson itself.

Instead of "It doesn't feel good when you do that," try "I've been wondering what it would feel like if you did it this way".

Instead of "You go too fast," try "I think if we go slower, you might be able to give me an even bigger orgasm."

The suggestions don't have to be verbal. Grabbing your partner's hand and placing it where you want it, along with a heartfelt moan can be a blameless, shameless step in the right direction.

The Closed Door
This position is similar to the missionary in that both people are lying down face-to-face, and the man is on top. The difference, however and what makes this an advanced position is that the woman will keep her legs shut tightly the entire time. The man's penis can be inserted while her legs are open and then once it is in, she will close her legs. What this does is constrict her vagina and make the canal tighter for the man's penis. In addition to this, if she is aroused her vagina will be engorged and the canal will be tighter already. Because of this, the man's penis will be hugged closely as it slides in and out of her and this will make for extra pleasure for him.

The Lap Dance
This next position is another that is best for male pleasure and the male orgasm. This position requires strength on the part of the man and the woman and is quite an athletic position, but

this is why it is called an advanced sex position. Be careful when trying this one.

To get into position, the man will sit upright in a comfortable chair or on the edge of a bed with his feet planted on the floor. The woman will climb onto his lap and wrap her legs around behind the man or stick them straight out past him. Then, the man can insert his penis into the woman's vagina. From here, the woman will lean back until she is lying straight back, and her body is flat. While she does this, the man will have to hold onto her at her hips or her lower back, depending on your height variations. The man in this position will perform a combination of thrusting his hips into the woman from a seated position and pulling her onto his penis repeatedly. A high amount of upper body strength is required on the part of the man in this position. Place some pillows on the floor underneath the woman when trying this position, just in case. The woman can hold onto the man's arms for support as well here.

This position is great for the male's pleasure because it allows him to control the speed and depth of thrusting, and it allows for deep penetration, which will feel amazing on his penis.

The Genie Lamp
A woman is on all fours as a man takes her from behind. While performing what is commonly know as "doggie style" the man waits until the woman is getting close to climax. He reaches around her and places his hands just above her pubic bone. He rubs his hands in opposite directions. Because this area is incredibly sensitive for woman, the stimulation can reach much higher levels.

The G Force

The man sits on the bed. Facing the man, the woman mounts him guides his penis into her. Then, with her hand flat on the bed for support, she begins the lovemaking. If the man bends his knees, she has the option of bracing herself on the to gain better position to control the rhythm and pace. While she is rising and lowering herself, the man places a fist above the base of his penis (just below his belly button). As the woman moves up and down, her clitoris will be stimulated by her partner's fist.

Women

Milk the Man

This move requires some training. A woman needs to perform about 25-30 Kegel exercises a day. When she has worked her Pubococcygeus muscles to where she is able to isolate the inner, middle and outer muscles, she is ready for the "milk-the-man" technique.

The man lies on his back. The woman mounts him and straddles him she guides his penis inside of her. She then clenches her PC muscles in sequence, starting with the one that's closest to the entrance of the vagina. This will be an experience that the man has not only experienced before, but didn't even know was possible!

Multiple-Male!-Orgasms

Whenever a man has an orgasm, it's followed by a refractory period, during which he can't become erect again. For Some men, this might last minutes, for others it might last days. What most men don't know is that the release of sperm and their orgasm can be separated.

When a man is about to ejaculate, press your middle firmly on the perineum (the ridge between the testicles and the anus). This will cut of the flow of semen while he has his orgasm. After the orgasm, he will find that he is immediately ready to go again.

The P-Spot

While pleasuring a man, he can be easily stimulated by massaging his prostate. This can be done externally, by rubbing the perineum (the ridge between the testicles and the anus) or internally but wetting a finger with lube and slowly massaging the outer rectum. This area is rich with nerve ending and can create immense please. Slowly insert the finger (short nails please) only a little bit, wait for the sphincter to relax before proceeding further.

The best way to massage the prostate is with the finger inside the anus, massaging what will feel like a walnut-sized sack (in the direction of the belly button). For the man with an adventurous spirit, a curved dildo can also be used to stimulate him. While this can be an incredibly gratifying experience for the man, it's important to know before hand that he is comfortable with it.

CHAPTER 8:

ORAL SEX

Oral Sex for Men by Women

When giving oral sex to a man, this involves the mouth of her partner stimulating his erogenous zones like his penis, his testicles, and his anus. When it comes to the man's penis, there are multiple ways that you can give oral sex.

The one main thing to note is whether the penis is uncircumcised versus circumcised. If the man's penis is uncircumcised, you will need to pull back the foreskin in order to expose the head of his penis. The good thing about this, though, is that his penis will be more sensitive than a non-circumcised penis underneath the foreskin, and this will make your oral sex feel amazing for him.

When giving oral sex to a man, you can use your mouth to stimulate his penis. While you do this, you can use your hands to please him in other areas like his testicles or his anus, whatever he likes. As you do it, he can communicate to you by telling you what he likes in terms of speed and pressure.

Guys love to get blow jobs because it usually doesn't involve much work on their end. The female mouth is also usually hotter than the vagina and is therefore more pleasurable for most guys. Plus, there's the 'swallowing' situation which a lot of guys find incredibly hot.

So how exactly can you provide the best oral sex possible? Here's what you should keep in mind when going down on your man.

Find the Most Comfortable Position for You

Guys have no problem of getting a blow job sitting down, standing up or lying down – they're all good with that as long as you'll have your mouth wrapped around their shaft. What's important here is that YOU (the female) find the most comfortable position for yourself; otherwise you won't last long in giving him fellatio. As most women will say, the most comfortable position would be on the bed with your man lying down. This way, your knees and elbows will be resting on something soft, keeping you comfortable and therefore more likely to linger on his erection. Once you manage to find the perfect position, you'll have more fun playing with his penis.

Get It Really Wet

Make sure the penis gets *really* wet; otherwise it won't be an enjoyable session. Obviously, saliva would be the main thing used as a lubricant. However, if you're partial to a little bit of flavor, then edible oils would be the perfect accompaniment for the oral pleasure. You'll find that there are literally dozens of possible flavors out on the market today so you won't have any problems finding one that works best for your needs.

Rhythm and Pace

The whole point of a blow job is to simulate penile-vaginal intercourse which means that you don't have to go fast and furious from the get go. Instead, use different speeds, pace, and depth so that your lover doesn't know what to expect next. It's perfectly OK to go slow first and then hit a fast pace and then go slow again. There's no specific speed or count – just follow your mood as well as pay attention to the signals of your partner.

Hardness May Vary
According to experts, it's not necessary for an erection to stay hard all through the fellatio. In fact, hardness may peak and ebb during the process so don't worry too much if your man gets a little softer during the oral game.

Look (And Sound) Like You're Really Enjoying It
This is perhaps one of the biggest turn-ons for most guys. The simple knowledge that YOU are enjoying having their cock in your mouth definitely kicks up the libido for the men. Now, there are lots of ways to show that you're enjoying what you're doing starting with eye contact. Look him in the eyes while giving a blow job, punctuated by moans and slurping. Think of it as ice cream and that you want to take your time enjoying the frozen delight before going to the main dish. Do NOT underrate moaning since a lot of guys love this, especially since the vibration in your throat provides additional stimulation to the shaft, thereby boosting the pleasure.

Take Your Time
Unless time is really of the essence – it's really not a good idea to rush a blow job. Believe us – a guy would like to enjoy every second of the experience and for most ladies – they enjoy the power of having the guy at their mercy. Although oral sex is in itself, a form of sex – it can also be a prelude to the real thing. Therefore, most women should treat is as a foreplay, taking their time, teasing, and giving as much attention as possible to the penis. Remember the illustration given above? Make sure to hit all the important spots, paying particular attention to the most sensitive points for the man. Use your tongue, lips, and mouth together, employing a sucking motion that can really get him moaning.

Teeth or Not to Teeth

This one's a little difficult to gauge. Some guys have no issue with the teeth getting some action during a blow job while others are very wary of it. After all, all guys are a little afraid of their Johnson getting cut off. For the sake of safety however, women are advised NOT to scrape the penis with their teeth since this can cause problems in the bedroom. A nip or a nibble can be acceptable provided that you test the water first. If he doesn't seem to like it, then simply don't do it again.

Smooth and Slow Technique

The smooth and slow technique refers largely to how you initiate the oral sex. There are lots of ways to start and for some men; this is definitely one of the most stimulating techniques. The process is to simply hold the base of his shaft firmly, pop open your lips a little bit and then slowly push the shaft inwards, making sure that the underside of the penis grazes the tongue. Go slow – one inch at a time while maintaining eye contact if possible. You can also try moaning while you do this to give that extra vibration to the penis.

This technique introduces heat to the shaft in one pleasurable inch at a time, somehow prolonging the experience and allowing the male to really appreciate the blowjob. An added bonus here is how the mouth slowly expands to accommodate the width of the penis – pretty much like a slow entry of the vagina. Go as deep as you can and hold the position for a few seconds before slowly retracting again, ensuring that the tongue grazes the bottom of the shaft one inch at a time.

Lip Stick Technique

The lip stick technique is more of foreplay to fellatio. It consists of using the penis as a lipstick by swiping it on the edge of your mouth. At the same time, this helps with lubrication so that the shaft will get in easier – not to mention hotter. The precum is also an excellent lubricant and for most men, licking it off gets them really turned on. You'll find that the lipstick technique also helps stimulate the underside of the penis which is the most sensitive part of the organ. Try a swipe and pop motion that offers a variety of pressure for the male.

Lick and Loves
Licking the penis is also an excellent way of playing during oral sex. Licks can be done in one long stroke or a few small strokes. There's no way inducing orgasm with tongue play, but it is an excellent way of boosting the male libido and teasing him until he goes crazy. Don't forget to lick the edges of the mushroom head where the nerve endings are concentrated.

Hot and Cold
Playing with heat and cold can also steadily increases the pleasure for most males. Some women like to expose the penis to the heat of their mouth and then put ice inside so that there's a rapid change to a cold temperature. The change makes the penis more sensitive and produces a different level of pleasure for the male. Unfortunately, it's not exactly a spontaneous event and may leave some awkward pauses in between the blow job. When done playfully however, you'll find that this works wonderfully. The hot and cold technique also works wonderfully if you include food play into the experience. For example, you can try putting ice cream on the penis, allow it to melt a little and then put the whole thing inside the mouth. This produces a wonderful blend of temperature that can make most guys groan in pleasure.

Deep Throat
Not all women can perform an awesome deep throat so he will definitely be grateful with this particular item in your repertoire. Deep throat action consists of putting the whole penis in your mouth – usually from the tip all the way to the

roots. The action envelops the male penis completely in heat which is basically what happens when the member enters the vagina. However, many males note that deep throat is often better because the mouth is remarkably hotter than the vagina, therefore producing more intense pleasures.

Considering how the average penis is marginally longer and thicker than the throat, it's not uncommon for women to gag while doing this. The gag reflex is tough to fight and need to be adjusted to slowly; otherwise you might find yourself vomiting during the deed. Most women practice by using a penis-sized object to fit in their mouth. A dildo or even a banana will do pretty well for this need. Practice the technique as often as possible until you get it right. Don't worry about producing too much saliva – this is something you definitely won't be able to avoid while doing the real thing. Some techniques to help out include getting the right position (kneeling is a major turn on plus it's actually easier to breathe in this situation).

Play with Everything
Remember: oral sex isn't just oral sex. There are lots of points for a guy that can help increase the pleasure during sex. In fact, stimulating guys is usually easier than girls. Make sure to play with the balls and if you have no qualms, putting the balls inside the mouth is every bit as pleasurable as putting the penis inside the mouth.

Sucking, licking, and nipping are all welcome when it comes to the penis and most males appreciate all these level of attentions. Caressing the buttocks, the inside of the thighs, and various other body parts can also help boost the pleasure. Some men actually like it when the female inserts a finger inside his anus.

Pay Attention
Remember what Chris Rock once said about guys and sex. For the most part, a blow job will get a guy hard and ready to come. However, if you manage to do what he likes exactly how he likes them, then he COMES.

It's a whole different level of pleasure that can be the difference between backyard fireworks and 4th of July fireworks. Hence, you can be sure that ALL the techniques above will leave your man aroused, but some techniques will REALLY blow his mind in the sack. PAY ATTENTION to his responses.

Which parts does he moan or what actions do you do that makes him grip and shudder under you?

Find out what he likes and incorporate more of those moves into your blow job to give your boyfriend the best possible oral sex he's ever had!

Positions
When it comes to oral sex for a man, there is a little-known secret. This secret is in the testicles and knowing how to use them to your advantage when giving him oral pleasure. The oral sex position described here uses this technique to add to the pleasure of a blow job.

Kneeling
This position is done when the man is standing up, and the woman is on her knees in front of him, giving him oral sex. While the woman is kneeling in front of the man and giving him oral sex, she can use one of her hands to hold onto his testicles and gently massage them. She will begin to stroke them softly as they will be very sensitive to the touch.

By holding them and very lightly pulling them towards her, this will drive him crazy as the stimulation of both his penis and his testicles at the same time will make it hard for him not to finish right then and there. The warmth and moisture of a mouth around his penis, along with his testicles being gently rubbed, will send him flying into the land of orgasmic bliss.

Oral Sex for Women by Men

When giving oral sex to a woman, this involves the mouth of her partner stimulating her erogenous zones, including her clitoris, her labia and her anus. As you learned earlier in this book, a woman can orgasm from two main places-the clitoris and the G-Spot. Since you are not able to stimulate the G-Spot with your mouth, oral sex involves the clitoris. Stimulating the clitoris with your tongue is the best way to give oral sex to a woman.

The best way to do this is to gently move your tongue around the clitoris and the vulva area. By starting out slowly and increasing speed gradually, this will get the woman's pleasure increasing at a steady state, which is the best way to make her reach orgasm. While you do this, you could touch her in other places like her vagina by inserting a finger. Some women enjoy the combination of these different types of pleasure.

If you want to give a woman orgasm every time, the best way to do it is through oral sex. There's nothing quite like it – especially if you get your technique polished to almost perfect. Unfortunately, most men do not perform oral sex too well and have a hard time committing to the activity. Here are some tips if you want to WOW her with your mouth:

Get Her Comfortable

Receiving oral sex for men is easy – not so for women. The position isn't exactly comfortable which is why it's important if you give her time to *really* get into position. Possibly the most comfortable position for oral sex would be lying down with pillows piled high under her pelvis. This tilts up the vagina and allows for a large opening, thereby giving you lots of room to work. In this position, guys also get lots of control and comfort so that they can play as much as they want.

Lick and Suck

Biting or nipping may be good for some guys receiving oral pleasure, but it's always a negative for the girls. Feel free to suck and lick as much as you want, but never let her feel the teeth because it will definitely bring her out of the moment.

Play with the Lips

The lips or labia is wonderfully sensitive, especially when it comes to light pressure. Using the edge of your tongue on this body part will definitely send shiver down her spine, especially if you follow up with a good and long hard suck.

Locate the Clitoris

Know where the clitoris is located and have fun with it. Note though that the clitoris shouldn't receive all your attention. Remember that in this position, you have access to both the clitoris and the U-Spot which is that sensitive plump flesh just a few centimes below the clitoris.

Rotating Stimulation

There's such a thing called rotating orgasm that basically talks about stimulating all the female 'spots' one after the other in a rotating fashion. According to some women, this would produce the most intense orgasm possible, unlike anything women have ever had. Unfortunately, this is mainly a theory rather than a proven fact since the technique used to achieve this is difficult to perfect.

During oral sex however, males are given lots of opportunity to hit the spots and induce orgasm. If you're not a fan of giving oral sex to the female and want her to orgasm as quickly as possible, it's a good idea to perform the act hitting as many spots as possible. For example, while stimulating the clitoris and U-Spot with your mouth, you can insert two fingers in the vagina to work on the A-Spot. While doing this, another hand can be used to stimulate the K-Spot – effectively allowing you to hit 4 important erogenous zones all the same time. Do this alternately or simultaneously, changing in pace, depth, and power in order to trigger a powerful and quick orgasm.

Listen and Learn

If you're not getting encouragement – either verbal or physical – you're probably not doing it right. Most women would moan or do something that tells you you're hitting the right spots. There are also instances when she'll grab the guy's hair and direct the movement of the lips and mouth, silently telling him where to go and which part to focus on. The tilting and shifting of the pelvis is also indicative of this particular need. Make sure to pay attention to these changes so you'll be able to fully give her the orgasm she wants or needs.

Not Just the Mouth

Note that oral sex isn't completely oral. In the same way the women use their fingers when giving a blow job, men can also use their fingers during oral sex. In fact, it's usually a better idea since their fingers can enter and stretch the vagina in such a way that men can stimulate two important points all at once: the clitoris and the A-Spot. If men are particularly good, they can also hit the U-Spot and the K-Spot at the same time.

Positions

There are many positions in which you can give oral sex to a woman. In this section, I will introduce one of these such positions that will be sure to give the woman great pleasure.

The Kivin

If you are a woman and your partner give you oral sex that feels nice, but that just doesn't quite push you to orgasm, this position may be perfect for you. Sometimes it is hard for the person giving a woman oral sex by stimulating her clitoris with their tongue to keep their tongue moving up and down fast enough to make the woman reach the type of clitoral orgasm that she would reach with fingers instead. The way to make this easier is with the following position.

Kivin is a position that allows a person to orally please a woman with a greater chance of helping her to reach orgasm than the traditional position of the head between her legs that most people are used to.

To get into this position, the man will have his partner lie on her back. He will then position himself lying perpendicular to her body, his head close to her vulva. Begin to touch her clitoris with your tongue and lips, gently moving your tongue back and forth over top of it. Turn your head to the side every once in a while, to see her face change as she is pleased. Move your tongue in small circles or use your lips to suck on her clitoris. Using your free hand, you can also reach up to her breasts and massage her nipples.

Giving her oral sex in this position places his tongue over her clitoris moving in a side-to-side motion, rather than an up and down motion and will give her greater pleasure because it allows his tongue to move over her clitoris at its most exposed angle. Trying it this way, she is sure to feel clitoral pleasure and will be likely to be able to reach orgasm.

CHAPTER 9:

ANAL SEX

A nal sex is something that not everyone has had experience with. It has the potential to provide you and your partner with very great pleasure if you know how to safely and comfortably engage in this type of sex. In this chapter, I will explain how you can safely have anal sex and how you can begin to use it to your advantage in order to experience pleasure like never before.

Anal Tips for Beginners

This collection of tips is carefully selected to help increase your pleasuring during anal, as well as protect you from any potential tearing or damage. It is recommended that you use these tips if you have never tried anal before, as they will help you build up to it and have a more enjoyable, and safe, experience.

Lubricate

Unlike the vagina, the anus does not lubricate itself naturally. Therefore, you have to use lubricant. There are many on the market that are warming, as well as some that are actually intended to help relax the muscles and make anal a more enjoyable experience for the lady. You should opt for a water-based lubricant of your choice.

Relax
As the lady, you really want to make sure you relax your muscles and take deep breaths. Go slow and take care not to tense up out of fear. In order to help reduce tensing up due to fear, make sure you follow the next step carefully.

Start Small
Especially if you are brand new to anal, as in an anal virgin, you will want to start very small. Using plenty of lube, and a small toy or his pinky finger, he can gently work his way into your bum and help you relax the muscles. He should move slowly and at your discretion, to ensure you are prepared for every step.

Go Slow
Aside from working your way up slowly, all movements should be slow as well. Once you're used to it, and have more confidence in the experience, you can start going faster. But every single anal experience should start with slow movements and shallow penetration. From there, he can choose how deep and quick he will go, based on how she feels.

Communicate
This is the one time you especially want to communicate well during sex. The lady should always be telling the gentleman if what he is doing is okay, and he should not be doing anything she doesn't like or that hurts her. You can even enforce a safe word that means you stop completely if one party is not enjoying themselves or is hurt by it.

Use Additional Stimulation
Anal feels a lot better for a lady if she is being stimulated beyond just through the butt. Rubbing her clitoris and nibbling on her upper shoulders or neck can greatly enhance her experience.

As well, having her focus on a pleasurable stimulation taking place elsewhere on her body can help her further relax her muscles and enjoy the experience.

Don't Go from Butt to Vagina
Never go from butt to vagina. Whether it is a finger, his penis, or a toy, nothing should ever penetrate the anus and then the vagina. This can lead to infections that are not enjoyable for anyone.

If You Absolutely Hate It, Stop
The first time or two can be extremely unenjoyable for the female, but eventually it can start feeling better. However, that being said, it should be noticeably better with each experience. If it is clearly not getting better, or it is getting worse, and one or both aren't enjoying it, then stop. You don't need to do it just because! Sex should always be fun and pleasurable for both lovers involved.

Kama Sutra Positions for Anal Sex
The following positions are great for people who are new to anal sex and would like to try some of the simpler positions in order to get used to the feeling of anal sex. These positions are straight from the Kama Sutra, or slight variations of Kama Sutra positions in order to make the optimized for anal sex.

Oral with Anal Stimulation
This first position is not involving anal penetration with a penis but is a great introduction to anal play. This position is done when a woman is giving a man oral sex. The man stands up and the woman is on her knees in front of him, giving him oral sex. She will then reach around behind the man's buttocks and stimulate his anus with her finger.

She can move her finger around the outside of his anus, stimulating the sensitive skin there which will make him feel immense amounts of pleasure. Giving oral sex and stimulating his anus at the same time will make it virtually impossible for him not to orgasm very quickly.

The Curled Angel
This is a Kama Sutra position that is written as a position to be performed with vaginal sex, but it can also be done as an anal sex position. This position involves the man and woman lying down on their sides, the man behind the woman. Both of them are facing the same direction, so the curve of their hips places the man's penis at the perfect point for anal penetration. In this position, the man and woman can grind their hips into each other, and it is a team effort in terms of control.

The Clip
In this position, the man lies back on the bed with his knees bent and his feet planted on the bed. The woman straddles the man and inserts his penis into her anus. In this position, she can lean forward onto the man's bent knees for support, and she is able to control the depth and speed of penetration. The man can hold onto the woman's buttocks and guide her movements as well.

The Snake
This position is a good one to try when you have a little bit of experience with anal sex but are not ready to try anything too extreme just yet. The person receiving anal penetration in this position takes a passive role and can just focus on relaxing and enjoying the pleasure rather than having to contort into some type of acrobatic formation.

To begin, the woman will lie face down on the bed, and her partner will lie on top of her, supporting himself with his arms.

From here, the woman will arch her back a bit to make her pleasure zones as accessible as possible for penetration. Now, the man will slowly slide his penis into her anus. Here, the woman can enjoy the pleasure ride her partner takes her on, without having to do anything herself. She is able to enjoy these moments where the focus is all on her!

Pegging

There is another type of anal sex that can be had, which involves sex toys. It is quite common that a woman will penetrate her male partner anally while wearing a strap-on. This practice is called Pegging. Now that you know a little more about sex toys and anal sex, and how to ensure you are combining these two in a safe and sanitary way, you are ready to try Pegging. This can be done either by using a dildo placed in a strap-on that a woman is wearing or by using a double-ended dildo. Using a double-ended dildo will allow the woman to be pleasured at the same time as she is penetrating the man, as she will also be penetrated either vaginally or anally with the other end of the dildo. This type of dildo looks like any other, except that it has two identical ends.

Now that you are aware of the possibility of this type of practice, you can understand how any of these anal sex positions can be performed by either the man penetrating the woman anally with his penis or by the woman penetrating her partner anally using a dildo.

For men, anal sex is extremely pleasurable since their prostate is stimulated through anal penetration. The prostate is what has been referred to as the "male G-Spot."

CHAPTER 10:

ORGASM

Male Orgasm Basics

The male orgasm is something that most people have witnessed or seen if they have ever watched any sort of porn or heard about it in the media. The male orgasm is made out to be extremely simple and easy to achieve, but in this section, we are going to examine it in more detail and break it down into more specific parts.

To start, are you aware that there are different types of male orgasms? If you are a male, you are likely aware of this, but if you are a female, you may not be. The term *male orgasm* includes any and every type of orgasm that involves the male's genitals.

Orgasm and Ejaculation

Ejaculation and orgasm for males are actually two distinct events, even though they most often happen at the same time. This fact makes them often misunderstood, as many think that ejaculation is a sign of orgasm. If orgasm occurs and ejaculation happens at the same time, this is called an **ejaculatory orgasm.**

There is another type of orgasm, one that happens when ejaculation does not. As you likely guessed, this type is called a **non-ejaculatory orgasm.** This is sometimes called a *dry orgasm* as well, and this type is also very normal. A man can achieve orgasm without ejaculation, and this still counts as an orgasm.

The Prostate

Different types of orgasms are often only mentioned when it comes to female bodies, but men are also able to experience different types of orgasms that don't involve their penis. This is another reason why ejaculation does not necessarily signal orgasm.

One of the most sensitive male erogenous zones is the prostate. The prostate is full of pleasure-potential for a man. The prostate is accessed through the anus, and this is why anal play for men can be so enjoyable. For a man, exploring his prostate may be a new experience for him and he may be a little bit skeptical, especially since it involves the anus. Anal play can be for everyone and anyone, and it has the potential to make a man reach new levels of orgasmic pleasure. The prostate is a secret weapon of such intense pleasure that you would be doing your man a disservice if you did not help him explore it.

A man can begin to explore his prostate on his own if he is not quite comfortable doing it with a partner. He can begin by including it in his next masturbation session in order to give himself a little extra love. Once he experiences the prostate sensations and feels comfortable and full of excitement about this newly discovered area of his body, he can also try it with a partner and show them how to please him in this way.

How to Find the Prostate

To start your first prostate exploration, set the mood right first. Set yourself enough time, remove distractions and worries, and really allow yourself to get into the mood. Start by touching yourself and getting yourself turned on, maybe watch a porn video you enjoy or just let your mind wander. When you get to the point of being very horny, but you haven't let yourself reach orgasm yet, you are ready to explore your prostate.

The key to discovering anything involving the anus is lube. Make sure you have lots of lube and take deep, relaxing breaths as you explore your butt hole. Begin by teasing the area around the hole for a while, just feeling what it feels like if you never have before. Close your eyes and let your feelings guide you. Move your finger around the hole gently and slowly. Your butt hole will expand as you go, so do not worry. When you are ready, slide your finger into your anus slowly. Breathe deeply and relax into your pleasure. Take your exploration slowly and gently. To find your prostate, curve your finger towards the front of your body, and you will feel a soft, bumpy surface. This is the spot.

How to Stimulate the Prostate to Achieve Orgasm
Once you have found the prostate, you can begin to gently massage this area and let the sensations build. Keep going like this and find out what type of movements or pressure feels best. As you continue to stimulate it, let the pleasure build until the point of orgasm. When you are comfortable with this spot, try having your partner stimulate it for you. Having someone else's hands touch it for you will feel different than your own, and with your free hand, you can turn yourself and your partner on in other ways.

The prostate is sometimes referred to as the male G-Spot. It has many similar properties to the female G-Spot, such as the way that you can find it and the way in which it needs t to be stimulated in order to reach orgasm. We will learn about the female orgasm in the following section.

Female Orgasm Basics
In order to make a woman orgasm, you will need to know and understand the female body, including all of the places where, when stimulated, a woman will feel pleasure and maybe even orgasm. Whether you are a female yourself or you are a male

with a female partner, both sexes can benefit from learning more about the female body.

The Clitoris
There are two main spots from which a woman can orgasm. The first is the clitoris.

The clitoris is the place that many people know of as the "orgasm spot" of a woman's body. This is arguably the easiest way to give a woman an orgasm. The clitoris is located very close to the vagina. It is a small, bean-like structure that has many, many nerve endings, which is why it is so sensitive and can so easily lead to female pleasure.

How to Find the Clitoris
In order to find the clitoris, begin by placing a hand on the pelvic area, with the fingers towards the vagina. A woman can do this to herself, or a man can do this to find the woman's clitoris. Slowly move your hand downward, using your fingers to feel around. As you wrap your fingers underneath her, between her legs, feel around for a small lump-like structure. It is in a slightly different spot, covered by different amounts of layers and of different sizes on every woman, so explore around between the legs to find it. It will be towards the front of her body, right where her vaginal lips begin.

The clitoris has been compared to the male penis, and some even call it "the female penis." This is because it actually enlarges and becomes engorged when a woman is sexually aroused, similar to a male erection. For this reason, it is much easier to find the clitoris when a woman is sexually aroused. The clitoris is much larger than it appears from the outside and this is because it extends into a woman's body. Only a small part of the clitoris is located on the outside of the body. The larger size of the clitoris is the reason that there are so many nerve endings located within it, and the reason why stimulating it will lead to such intense pleasure.

How to Stimulate the Clitoris to Achieve Orgasm

Once you have found the clitoris, you will then be able to stimulate it in order to achieve orgasm. Begin by gently placing two fingers on it and putting a bit of pressure. Rub it by moving your fingers in small circles-making sure to be gentle. Continue to do this, and she should begin to get more aroused the more you do this. By rubbing the clitoris, you will be able to stimulate the entire clitoris, even the part of it that you cannot see, and this will cause the woman to start to become wet in her vaginal area in order for her body to prepare for sex.

The G-Spot

The G-Spot is a lesser-known spot than the clitoris, but it is possible for a woman to have extreme amounts of pleasure when this spot is stimulated. The reason that the G-Spot can give a woman intense pleasure is that it is actually connected to the clitoris. Inside the body, where the clitoris extends up into the woman, it meets the vagina, and this is the spot where the G-Spot is located. This thin wall between the clitoris and the inner vagina allows for the pressure and stimulation from sex to stimulate both spots. Therefore, one is essentially also stimulating the clitoris when they are pleasuring a woman's G-Spot.

How to Find the G-Spot

To find this spot, you will need to insert a finger into her vagina. It is best to try to find this spot after you stimulated the clitoris for a bit because then her vagina will have begun to get wet-as it lubricates itself to prepare for penetration. You can use this to your advantage because it will make penetration more enjoyable for her and will reduce the friction of the entire vaginal area in general. When the vagina becomes very wet, it can lubricate the entire vaginal area, including the clitoris, which will then make it easier to stimulate the clitoris as well. No friction means smooth gliding, which results in pleasure and no pain. When she is wet enough, slide a finger inside of her vagina while she is lying on her back (a woman can do this for herself too) and make a "come here" motion with your finger so that you are moving it towards her belly button. Feel around in this are and when you feel a bumpy or rough surface, this is the G-Spot. Just like the clitoris, the G-Spot is slightly different for every woman but they can all be in the same general area. The G-Spot will be of different sizes for different women, so be aware of this when trying to find it.

How to Stimulate the G-Spot to Achieve Orgasm
In order to give a woman pleasure by stimulating her G-Spot, you will need to press on it over and over again until she reaches orgasm. The G-Spot needs to receive continued and consistent stimulation in order for the pleasure to build enough for her to reach orgasm.

Since a woman can have two different types of orgasms, one from stimulating the clitoris and a different one from penetration or hitting the G-spot, this could be why a woman is able to reach orgasm during oral sex, or by having her clitoris stimulated, but has trouble actually reaching the same level of pleasure during penetrative sex. In many positions, the G-spot is not actually stimulated by the man's penis, and this can result in the woman having some amount of pleasure, but not enough to reach orgasm. For a great experience as a couple, knowing what makes the woman feel great is paramount.

For many people, when it comes to lovemaking, the orgasm isn't the cherry on top. It's the entire sundae. They treat foreplay and intercourse as if there were playing poker and if they play their cards right, they win the pot and cash those chips in for a mind-blowing, body quivering orgasm.

What if they don't climax? Well, then they treat the whole experience as though the won the pot only to discover the chips can't be cashed in. They're stuck with two handfuls of worthless plastic. Everyone can agree that orgasms feel amazing. It's a sure sign that all the elements in lovemaking came together perfectly to give that partner a moment of ecstasy.

As great as they are, it's a huge mistake to make that the goal of lovemaking, especially when practicing the Kama Sutra. When practicing the techniques, the experience shouldn't be judge on whether or not one or both partners experienced orgasms. In fact, they shouldn't even be basing it on how close they came to climaxing. Orgasms can be very elusive, especially for women. Sometimes it might take more time than they have. Sometimes thinking about it makes it difficult to actually have it. Sometimes, it doesn't happen because it just didn't happen.

The Kama Sutra is not a pass/fail approach sex. If anything, it's an independent study, where you are allowed to choose your own interests, explore at your own pace, and finish whenever you want (within reason). When it comes to becoming more connected through sex, it the foreplay and the intercourse that builds awareness, connectivity, and pleasure that is shared. Your orgasm is exactly that: yours. Your partner might be thrilled that you're having it, but it's not shared the same way you share affection, kissing and intercourse.

By taking one's mind off of getting or giving an orgasm, other thing become more memorable and ultimately more meaningful. Everything from a caress to a lick to switching up the angle of penetration can be judged for it's own merit instead of how much closer it brought someone to climax.

CHAPTER 11:

MESTRUAL CYCLE AND SEX

During a woman's younger years, she will get her period every month. Period is the casual term for menstruation, and it is how it will be referred to hereafter. Once a month, if a woman does not get pregnant, she will get her period, which involves the lining of her uterus being shed. This makes way for the possibility of pregnancy the next month, as the uterus will develop a new lignin over the month. A period usually lasts about a week and involves skin cells and blood being shed through the vagina. The reason for this is that there is extra skin and blood that accumulate in the uterus to prepare for a possible pregnancy, but it will only last for one month at a time.

Benefits and How it Affects Sex

If a woman is comfortable, there is no problem with her having sex during her period. There is nothing that says that a woman should not, and it will not hurt the man or the woman. As long as neither of them is afraid of blood, the only difference will be the mess that it will cause. Women actually tend to have a much higher sex drive during their periods and during the week leading up to it.

There are some benefits that come from having sex on your period. One of these benefits is that having sex while on your period can actually offer relief from the pain of period cramps. Period cramps can be very painful, and anything that makes them feel better is a welcome suggestion, especially when it feels as good as sex will. This result is because of the orgasm. The chemicals that are released in the brain make you feel happy and also have pain relief functions. The other reason is that an orgasm makes the uterus contract and then release. The release part of this will likely make a woman feel better than she did before in terms of cramps.

Another benefit of having an orgasm during your period is that it leads to the uterus contracting, which actually pushes the blood and uterus contents out faster, leading to a shorter period length. This also means that there is ample natural lubrication and that lubricant is not necessary during period sex.

Best Kama Sutra Positions to Try During Menstruation

A good way to have sex during menstruation is in the shower. This makes it so that there is not much cleanup involved, and the blood that gets on either of you will be able to be washed off right away. This is a cleaner and more comfortable alternative to having sex in bed and having to jump in the shower afterward. Additionally, shower sex is steamy (literally) and hot (literally) and can make for some very fun body-on-body action. Make sure the water is the perfect temperature and that you have a mat or something on the floor so you aren't slipping all over the place! Before you start any type of penetration in the water, make sure you use lots of waterproof lube because the water in the shower won't be enough of a lubricant for the inside of a vagina and will actually make for some painful friction. Let's avoid that; lube is your friend!

Standing Doggy Style

Standing Doggy Style is a position from the Kama Sutra with a twist. It is a good place to start with shower sex because it will make sure that you don't get sprayed in the face with a hot stream of water while you are trying to focus on having a blissful orgasm. Pleasurable for both parties, Doggy Style in the shower is a new take on an old favorite.

The man stands with his back to the running water with the woman standing in front of him, facing away from him. The woman then bends forward and can put her hands on the edge of the tub or the wall of the shower for support. The man slides his penis into her from behind, grabbing onto her hips for a deeper thrust, and then they are ready to go for it. This position has a good chance of the man being able to hit the woman's G-spot with his penis, so this position will be greatly enjoyed by the woman. The warmth and the wet environment of the shower are sure to make for an unforgettable sexual encounter.

Kama Sutra Shower Sex Position
This is another position to try in the shower. If you both are in the mood for a position that doesn't need you to focus too much on difficult positioning and holding yourselves up in a slippery shower, you can try the kneeling position. Have yourselves kneel on the floor of the shower, one person behind the other? From here, you can go in many different ways. You can use this position as foreplay as you both reach around to pleasure the other's genitals with your hands before you move to the bedroom together. You can also use this as foreplay before switching to another position for penetration in the shower. Or you can start penetration right away. For penetration, you will have to adjust each of your heights on your knees to line up your erection and her vagina to meet nicely for smooth penetration. This position is full of possibilities and is a very hot way to get you both in the mood for whatever is to come either in the shower or out of it.

Bouncy Chair

This is not a shower position, but it is a great position for having sex during your period. This is because it can be done on the floor so that you can more easily clean up afterward.

To get into this position, the man will get on his knees on the floor (on towels or sheets for ease of cleaning) and sit back on his heels. The woman will sit on his lap, facing him, and put his penis inside of her. She will keep her feet planted on the floor and use the balls of her feet to bounce herself up and down on the man's penis. This position is great because the woman is hovering over the floor and this will allow for most of the blood to land there instead of all over the bed or the man.

Things to Keep in Mind

There are a few things to keep in mind if you and your partner decide that you wish to have sex on your period.

Blood Stains

Ensure that before you begin, if you are going to have sex anywhere outside of the bathtub or the shower, that you put down a lot of towels or something that will be able to absorb the blood. If you get it on your white bed sheets, it will stain. Keep I mind as well that whatever towels you choose to lay down will also likely be stained, so be sure to choose those that you don't need to keep freshly white.

Self-Consciousness

Having sex during her period may make a woman feel self-conscious. Keeping this in mind is important as she may feel sensitive about her body or the amount of blood that is involved.

Sexually Transmitted Infections

One thing that is important to note is that there are some STIs that are transmitted through the blood. These are HIV or hepatitis. In order to stay safe, it is important to use condoms all the time, but especially when there will be blood involved during sex.

Tampons

Tampons that are forgotten about when having sex can cause a problem. If you were wearing a tampon before having sex, ensure that you remove it before a penis or fingers are inserted into the vagina. Otherwise, the tampon will need to be removed by a doctor.

You Can Still Get Pregnant

While the chances are lower during your period, you can still become impregnated during your period. It is difficult to say at what point your body will be ready to conceive during your period, so taking adequate precautions is necessary.

CONCLUSION

Thank you again for downloading this book! I hope you learned a lot! I hope this book was able to help you to incorporate your own creativity and unique desires into the techniques presented.

The next step is to grab your partner's hand and venture into the art of foreplay, emotional transparency and exploration of each other's sexual appetite!

By using some of the moves in this book, we hope you have been able to improve your bedroom experience and share a more romantically intimate relationship with each other.

This is the first step toward creating change in your life. Reconnecting with yourself, your partner and your place in the universal order, is the first step in a journey of one thousand miles. The destination is much less important than the journey. This is probably the most enduring theme of Kama Sutra. The quality of your journey is defined by your awareness of its beauty and the many details that make its progress delightful and joyful.

Being consciously, intentionally and mindfully engaged with our sexuality serves to hold together the universe by reinforcing the great love at its core. As a sexual being seeking a deeper and more fulfilling connection with your partner, you're also seeking a deeper and more fulfilling connection with the cosmos itself. Your part in the divine plan and in your divinely-gifted sexuality is part of what makes the universe an integrated whole. By learning to give sexuality the exalted and holy position in your life it deserves, you are becoming more attuned to what it means to be human.

By re-igniting the flame of desire between you, you will draw closer to one another than you'd ever believed possible, even at the beginning of your relationship. Sexuality is a spiritual reality, not just a physical one.

Make sure that if both parties are **not** on board for trying something new, or with sex altogether, that you stop. You always want to honor your spouse's wishes, by respecting what they say they don't want. Consent is very important when it comes to sex, and proceeding without consent can deeply damage the intimacy and trust experienced between lovers. Never do something that your spouse doesn't want to do, and never pressure them to feel like they should have to do it.

Thank you and good luck

~ 225 ~

www.ingramcontent.com/pod-product-compliance
Lightning Source LLC
Chambersburg PA
CBHW060317030426
42336CB00011B/1093